FOODALYTICS

A Data-Driven Approach To Discovering The Healthiest Foods

Nicholas J. Riebe
http://HaleGenic.com

HaleGenic Publishing

Published by HaleGenic Publishing, Minneapolis, Minnesota

Disclaimer

No part of this publication may be reproduced or transmitted in any form or by any means, mechanical or electronic, including photocopying or recording, or by any information storage and retrieval system, or transmitted by email without permission in writing from the publisher.

While all attempts have been made to verify the information provided in this publication, neither the author nor the publisher assumes any responsibility for errors, omissions, or contrary interpretations of the subject matter herein.

This book is for entertainment purposes only. The views expressed are those of the author alone, and should not be taken as expert instruction or commands. The reader is responsible for his or her own actions.

Adherence to all applicable laws and regulations, including international, federal, state and local, governing professional licensing, business practices, advertising and all other aspects of doing business in the US, Canada, or any other jurisdiction is the sole responsibility of the purchaser reader.

Neither the author nor the publisher assumes any responsibility or liability whatsoever on behalf of the purchaser or reader of these materials.

Any perceived slight of any individual or organization is purely unintentional.

ISBN 978-0-9997907-0-0 (paper)
Cover design by Mai C. Vang and Nicholas J. Riebe
Interior design by Kimberley Washington and Nicholas J. Riebe

Your Free Bonus

As a way of saying *thanks* for your purchase, I'm offering a free bonus that's exclusive to my book and blog readers.

Do you know what "The 3 Pillars of Health" are? These are the things that, deep down, we as humans all need to be successful at life. And if one pillar is weaker than the others, then we run the risk of them all crashing down.

If you're interested in discovering what these three pillars are and building a well-rounded life, then I recommend you visit my site so you can download your copy of *The 3 Pillars of Health*, which is an eight-page book that walks you through each of the pillars, and teaches you how to get them working together so you can be your best self. Visit the below link to receive instant access:

http://HaleGenic.com/3Pillars

THE 3 PILLARS OF HEALTH

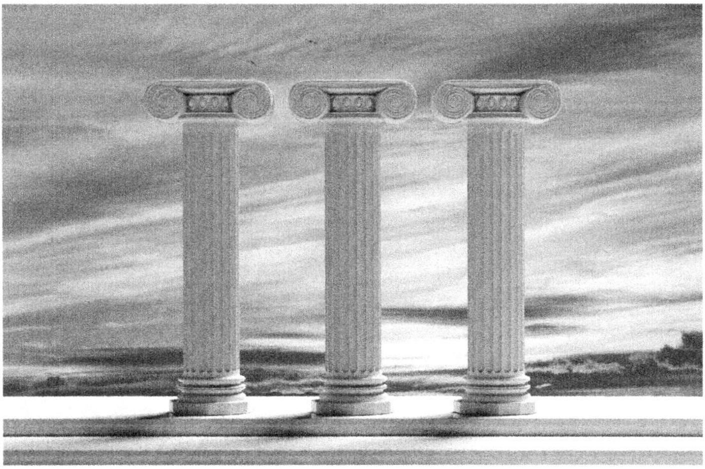

TABLE OF CONTENTS

INTRODUCTION

If I asked you what the healthiest foods are, what would you say? Kale? Spinach? Broccoli? While these foods are healthy, you'd be incorrect to assume they are the healthiest. In fact, broccoli isn't even in the top 25!

Everybody wants to eat healthy these days, but healthy eating becomes more of a challenge when you're balancing home cooking against social eating or the convenience of food delivery services. And then when you finally get a chance to focus on eating healthy, what foods should you choose?

What is a healthy food? Food with vitamins in it? Foods with more protein and less carbohydrates? Is it food that will help you lose weight? Is there any way to objectively sort out how healthy one food is compared to another?

I am an analyst by trade, and I've spent most of my career analyzing large amounts of data and extrapolating relevant information from it. This may sound boring to most, but to me, it's fun, like taking the scattered pieces of a puzzle and arranging them into artwork. So, when I made the resolution to determine the healthiest foods, it didn't come as a surprise that I took an analytical approach. Faced with measuring and evaluating the nutritional information of nearly 9,000 foods, my knowledge and understanding of data certainly came in handy.

I wrote *Foodalytics* for people who want to eat healthier and for those who may be already eating healthy but want to take things to the next level. This book will help you scientifically determine why a food like kale is good for you, its specific nutrients, how it compares to spinach and broccoli, and where, exactly, it lands within the healthiest food rankings.

With the abundance of processed foods today, it's easy to fall victim to not only food addictions, but also poor eating behaviors, like overeating and crash dieting. If you really want to be healthy for the rest of your life, you need to adopt a health philosophy that provides optimal energy, function, and defense mechanisms, as well as longevity. In order to do this, you must consistently choose to eat healthy foods at every meal, even if it means getting creative with things you don't find particularly tasty.

Perhaps you eat very little of a certain food group and need to start incorporating more of it in your diet. Maybe you're already eating well and maximizing nutritional intake is your prime directive. No matter where you are in your health journey, *Foodalytics* will always be your ultimate nutritional companion. This book is not a fad diet or a get-thin-quick scheme—rather, it's a guidebook to help you become healthier on the inside, as well as the outside. The next time you're faced with a nutritional decision between foods, worry not! Simply pick up this book to make the healthiest choice.

My Story

When I was growing up, I had no idea why it was important to eat healthy and exercise regularly. After all, I was just a kid and didn't think much about the subject of health, except maybe that being sick meant you weren't healthy and couldn't go out to play. For me, eating vegetables instead of sweets was just something your parents forced you to do. Maintaining a healthy weight was a foreign concept to me, as I was too busy running around, playing baseball, basketball, street hockey, or tag in the neighbors' yards.

I was never an obese child. In fact, I was always at the low end of the weight spectrum. My family and I ate the typical food pyramid diet: a large portion of meat and grains, some dairy, and some fruits and vegetables. Let's not forget the sweets group, either: a good dessert after dinner was standard for us, and it helped satisfy my sweet tooth. As long as my sister and I weren't eating too much junk food and were staying active, my parents were happy. Even back then, being thin was associated with being healthy.

When I was a teenager, my grandfather suffered from a massive stroke. The doctors put a stint in his carotid artery, and he came home from the hospital. After the stroke, though, he wasn't quite the same, and he died a few years later—just three days before my fifteenth birthday—at the age of 83. Although my grandfather's stroke was tragic to me, I never considered it as something I could be at risk for as an adult, nor did it provoke me to research what causes a stroke and how they could be prevented. I figured these diseases were merely caused by old age or genetic bad luck.

Fast forward eleven years to 2011, when I stumbled upon a two-hour video that shook up my thinking about food and health completely and changed the course of my life forever. The video was titled "Mark Sisson's Primal Life," starring Mark Sisson, the founder of the primal health movement. Mark walks viewers through the dangers of consuming processed food at any age, arguing that the nutritional choices you make, even in your youth, will directly impact the quality of your life in the future. For me, his most powerful message is how much nutrition people forego by choosing processed foods over whole food options. Refined carbohydrates (breads, pastas, and cereals) are especially poor choices, as they're merely high-energy, low-nutrient foods.

When I heard this, my jaw hit the floor. These foods had been a fundamental part of my diet for the last 25 years, and now I was being told I'd grown up eating one of the least nutritious foods out there! The video not only taught me how important it is to take a proactive approach to health, but also ignited a fire in me — a lifelong passion for discovering what it truly means to be healthy.

I began to wonder what would have happened if my grandfather had eaten better and been more active in his 50s into his 80s. What if he had rejected processed foods and refused to deviate from the farm fresh foods of his youth? Would he have been around longer to watch me grow up? How would my life have been different if he hadn't passed away when I was so young?

Two years into my own health journey, the unthinkable happened: my 92-year-old grandmother suffered a massive stroke and passed away merely a week later. It was one of the saddest moments of my life to see the most positive, happy, and kind person I'd ever known lying there during her final moments, unable to speak, eat, or even move. After her death, I knew deep down that something else was at play—something beyond genetics—and it gave me a newfound motivation for continuing to improve my health.

At this point, I became very grateful to have started down the path toward better health. The more I learned about it, the more certain I was that eating healthy was the key to reducing one's risk of suffering from the three leading causes of death: heart disease, stroke, and cancer. I want others to eat healthy as well so that, when they reach old age, they can go peacefully and their loved ones won't have to suffer through the same pain I experienced for both of my grandparents.

As I continued along my journey, I expanded my definition of health beyond just eating the right foods. I began increasing the quality of the food I was purchasing, improving my sleep and exercise, reducing stress, and also limiting my exposure to environmental hazards and toxins.

Today, I run a blog at HaleGenic.com where I document my experiments and push the envelope on all things related to health. *Foodalytics* is my first major contribution to the health community and truly is one of a kind. A fact-based analysis of what really makes a food healthy, this book will be a great companion as you continue your own health journey.

PART I

THE DEFINITION OF A HEALTHY FOOD

1

WHAT IS A NUTRIENT?

"A healthy outside starts from the inside."

—ROBERT URICH

The first step to understanding what makes a food healthy is to determine *what* is in it that is beneficial to the human body. The primary reason we eat food is for the nutrition and energy it provides. Nutrients are the absorbable elements of food necessary for life, and all foods contain varying degrees of these five nutrient types:

- Macronutrients
- Micronutrients
- Phytonutrients
- Fiber
- Water

The above elements are considered *essential nutrients* because they cannot be synthesized in sufficient quantities by the body and must come from dietary sources.

MACRONUTRIENTS

Macronutrients are comprised of the three nutrient types you read about most: fats, proteins, and carbohydrates. You often hear people say things like, "reduce your fat intake," "eat more protein," or "only eat carbs on workout days." You've probably also heard, "fat makes you fat," or the opposite: "at least 50% of your energy should come from healthy fats."

Generally speaking, all three macronutrients are important and it's nearly impossible to survive without them. Regardless of what you believe or subscribe to, your ideal macronutrient ratios ultimately depend on how your body responds to each type and your activity levels.

Fat

Fat is an important macronutrient that plays an integral part in the sustainment of human life. It provides protection to our vital organs, aids with body temperature regulation, gives us energy, and allows certain soluble vitamins to be dissolved into the body (vitamins A, D, E, and K, which are all necessary for optimal health).

Fats are made of molecules called triglycerides, which consist of two main components: glycerol and fatty acids. The specific glycerol to fatty acid ratio is what determines whether a fat will be a solid or liquid, the likelihood of rancidity, and if the fat is good or bad for you. Fat has historically gotten a bad rap, but the latest research shows it's not the amount of fat you consume that matters, but the kind.

There are two main categories of fats: saturated and unsaturated. Within unsaturated fats, there are three subtypes: monounsaturated, polyunsaturated, and trans. Trans-fats have officially been established to "no longer be safe"[1] by the FDA, yet the FDA still allows manufacturers to list 0 grams of trans-fat on the label—even if it has up to 0.5 grams per serving! The good news is you can easily tell if a food has trans-fat by doing a little investigative work. If it has "partially hydrogenated" in the ingredients list, the food has trans-fat and should be avoided.

Humans can synthesize saturated fats and some monounsaturated fats, but they lack the necessary enzymes to insert a double bond at the n-3 and n-6 positions of a polyunsaturated molecule. In other words, there are two essential fats which cannot be synthesized by the body: omega-3 and omega-6. These are two very popular fats you might have heard of before, but if not, that's okay—you'll learn more about them in Chapter 3.

Complications may arise from diets that include little to no fat intake, including weakening of the bones, kidney failure, and damage to the immune system. At extremely low fat intakes, you could suffer from a form of malnourishment called rabbit starvation. This unique form of poisoning got its name from indigenous peoples whose diets often consisted solely of rabbit meat, which is very lean, and who would end up suffering from extreme fat hunger.

Symptoms of rabbit starvation include diarrhea, headache, and physical weakness, not to mention an overall feeling of dissatisfaction, even after eating until their stomachs are distended—a symptom we still see often in malnourished children in third-world countries. Other problems that stem from lack of fat intake may include hair loss, brittle nails, and even premature death.

Protein

Protein's primary responsibility, at the cellular level, is to execute tasks directed by nucleic acids (think DNA and RNA). Each of our cells contains thousands of different proteins with important directives ranging from providing structural components for cells and tissues to defending against infection via antibodies.

Inadequate protein and amino acid intakes may lead to the catabolism (destructive metabolism) of muscles, while chronically low intake levels can lead to serious consequences, such as the breakdown of internal organs. This is why it's important for vegans to look for non-meat protein sources.

Protein is found in the following food groups: meat and seafood, vegetables (like spirulina), dairy and egg products, legumes, and grains. Like many food sourcing, protein doesn't come without it's warnings and controversies:

1. **Meat and seafood.** Sourcing has been a hot topic in the recent years, resulting in a greater emphasis on locally-sourced, free-range, and organic products.

2. **Dairy and egg products.** Scientists continue to go back and forth on whether eggs and milk are good or bad for you.

3. **Legumes.** Some researchers caution legume intake due to the presence of lectin in beans and phytoestrogens in soy products.

4. **Grains.** Quinoa is a popular grain that contains protein, however, evidence exists that the saponins in quinoa might be toxic to the body.

I don't say this to scare you, but to encourage you to make smart choices and do your own research when evaluating protein sources. The bottom line is that protein is a critical macronutrient and an important building block of life, representing a large piece in the big health puzzle.

Carbohydrate

The last of the macronutrients is carbohydrates, sugars with the primary purpose of providing energy to the body's tissues and cells. Broken down into two main classes, carbohydrates are comprised of *simple carbohydrates* (monosaccharides and disaccharides) and *complex carbohydrates* (polysaccharides and oligosaccharides).

All carbohydrate classes contain monosaccharides, the simplest form of sugar, and when a hydrogen atom is removed from this molecule, energy is produced. Glucose and fructose are the most common forms, and when joined together, two monosaccharides form a disaccharide (commonly referred to as table sugar or sucrose). Polysaccharides can be broken down into two groups: structural and storage. A storage polysaccharide is the carbohydrate listed on nutrition labels.

If you consume fat and protein but few carbohydrates, your body begins a natural process called *ketogenesis*, in which the body converts fat into energy (consuming zero carbs, however, although nearly impossible to do, is not recommended and can become problematic). Even the Inuit, known for a diet of nearly 100% fat and protein, still consumed small amounts of plants from willow and spruce leaves, which helped them avoid diseases caused by a vitamin C deficiency, like rickets and scurvy.

MICRONUTRIENTS

Vitamins

A vitamin is simply any organic chemical compound required in limited amounts by an organism. Because vitamins cannot be synthesized by the body in sufficient quantities, they are also considered *essential*. Even though your body can make its own vitamin D and K, it is unable to produce enough. This is why we must look to outside sources, like foods and supplements, to reach the recommended daily intake levels for essential vitamins.

Vitamins support cellular functions, aid in growth and development, optimize the immune system, increase energy levels, and regulate body metabolism. Although deficiencies are rare, the effects can be serious. Over time, inadequate vitamin intakes can lead to chronic health problems, such as heart disease, cancer, and osteoporosis.

*Common Vitamins**

1. Vitamin A
2. Thiamine (Vitamin B1)
3. Riboflavin (Vitamin B2)
4. Niacin (Vitamin B3)
5. Pantothenic Acid (Vitamin B5)
6. Vitamin B6
7. Biotin (Vitamin B7)
8. Vitamin B12 (cobalamin or methylcobalamin)
9. Vitamin C
10. Vitamin D
11. Vitamin E
12. Vitamin K1
13. Vitamin K2
14. Folate
15. Choline

Like all nutrients, we must pay attention to quality when we source our daily vitamins. For example, it's generally better to get vitamin C from a fresh bell pepper than a pill, but the sourcing of the pepper, pill, and desired quantity all need to be considered. In the case of Vitamin C, supplements are often derived from ascorbic acid (a synthetic form of vitamin C that's an isolated part of the whole), which is commonly sourced from corn starch, corn sugar, or rice starch, rather than whole foods. Supplements sourced from whole foods and do not contain ascorbic acid, ascorbates, or additives exist, but are often expensive and difficult to find.

Minerals

Minerals are inorganic compounds that come from the earth and make up roughly 4% of the human body. They play an important role in building strong bones and teeth, controlling nerve and muscular function, and regulating our heartbeat. Additionally, minerals produce enzymes and hormones in the body, help maintain proper blood circulation, protect cellular integrity, and manage energy levels.

We typically ingest minerals by consuming foods grown in nutrient-rich soils. During the last 100 years, however, mineral levels have been depleted by over 85% in North American soils. According to the United Nations' 1992 Earth Summit Report, this is a result of intensive industrial agriculture focused on breeding fruits and vegetables that are bigger, better looking, and have longer shelf lives. Now more than ever before, it is crucial we choose mineral-dense foods and consider supplementation, so we can meet the daily recommended amounts for minerals.

There are two basic types of minerals: *macro* and *trace*. The body needs relatively large amounts of macro minerals (sometimes called *major minerals*) and low amounts of trace minerals.

Common macro minerals and trace minerals, include:

*Macro Minerals**

1. Calcium
2. Magnesium
3. Potassium
4. Sodium
5. Phosphorus
6. Chloride
7. Sulfur

*Trace Minerals**

1. Iron
2. Zinc
3. Selenium
4. Copper
5. Manganese
6. Iodine
7. Chromium
8. Cobalt
9. Fluoride

PHYTONUTRIENTS

Phytonutrients are health-promoting compounds found in both vegetables and fruits, initially produced to help plants protect themselves from fungi, germs, and bugs. Phytonutrients aren't necessary for human survival, but they play an important role in preventing disease and ensuring our bodies are functioning at optimum levels.

---

*A detailed explanation of the benefits and required amounts of each vitamin, and many of the macro and trace minerals can be found in Chapter 3.

Phytonutrients are best known for their anti-inflammatory and antioxidant properties, as well as the role they play in liver health. To date, over 25,000 phytonutrients have been discovered—and scientists are discovering more each day—but only a handful are well understood at this time.

Phytonutrients are classified into groups, including the carotenoid group, which consists of five important phytonutrients: alpha-carotene, beta-carotene, beta-cryptoxanthin, lutein and zeaxanthin, and lycopene. All five are on my list of the most essential nutrients (see Chapter 3) and are a significant part of my nutritional analysis. Other notable phytonutrient groups include flavonoids (the largest group with over 6,000 types), anthocyanins, polyphenols, glucosinolates, phytoestrogens, and resveratrol.

One of the major reasons processed foods fail to measure up to the nutritional quality and complexity of whole foods is because they are missing phytonutrients. This is why incorporating whole, phytonutrient-rich foods into our diets is important and a relatively easy way to take your health to the next level.

FIBER

Fiber is the indigestible part of a plant that helps move food through the body. It plays a vital role in overall digestive health and is found in fruits, vegetables, legumes, and grains. Doctors recommend men and women consume between 30-38 grams and 21-25 grams, respectively, of fiber each day.

There are two types of fiber: soluble and insoluble. Soluble fiber helps the body remove LDL cholesterol molecules and regulate blood sugar by slowing the absorption of glycogen. Insoluble fiber, on the other hand, passes through the body and remains relatively intact. It is responsible for increasing the bulk of your stools and reducing the instance of bowel-related problems, such as constipation, hemorrhoids, and loose stools (fecal incontinence). Both types of fiber play a role in satiation, helping you feel full while staving off hunger, and are effective solutions for weight management.

Consuming too much fiber, however, can cause bloating, cramps, abdominal pain, gas, and constipation. Interestingly enough, constipation is a symptom resulting from both too low and too high of fiber intake. If you consume too much fiber, it becomes difficult for the bulk to move through your system, but consume too little and your body will have a difficult time moving food through the digestive tract. In the instance of excess fiber, drinking more water can help. On the other hand, those low in fiber should work on increasing their fiber intake.

WATER

You've probably heard it all your life: the human body is made of over 70% water. Why is water so prevalent in the human body? Water helps remove waste and toxins, aids in digestion, and prevents the body from suffering from one of the most underrated conditions: dehydration. Without water, life on Earth would not exist. It is the single most essential nutrient and our planet's most valuable natural resource.

It is important to pay attention to your daily water intake. If you do not drink adequate amounts of water every day, you can suffer from dehydration and possibly death. Although this book is about the healthiest foods, it's water that makes any of this possible. After all, a person can live up to three weeks without food, but only three days without water!

So what are you waiting for? Go grab a glass and take a big gulp before moving on to the next chapter.

2

WHAT MAKES ONE FOOD HEALTHIER THAN ANOTHER?

"The food you eat can be either the safest and most powerful form of medicine or the slowest form of poison."

—*DR. ANN WIGMORE*

Making food choices today is more difficult than ever due to the overwhelming number of unhealthy options available. What makes matters worse is that many of these foods try to appear healthy by playing on our fears of having high cholesterol, high blood pressure, and getting fat. If sawdust was labeled as all-natural, low-sodium, low-cholesterol, and fat-free, would you buy it? I didn't think so. An unhealthy food is an unhealthy food, no matter how you dress it up.

Now, I'm not saying foods that are advertised as healthy are bad for you, but read your food labels and use caution when the packaging uses vague language. Even once we master the art of reading food labels and a list of ingredients, however, we still need to know which foods to choose and how to measure their differences.

In Chapter 1, you learned what a nutrient is. With this information in mind, let's dive into the three main nutritional factors that matter most when comparing foods: nutrient density, nutrient diversity, and nutrient synergy.

1. NUTRIENT DENSITY

A food that is nutrient dense has a high amount of nutrients per serving or per calorie consumed. If you ate one serving of salmon and received a total of 30 units of nutrition and then ate a brownie with only 2 units of nutrition, the serving of salmon would be 15 times more *nutrient dense* (nutritious) than the brownie.

With a finite number of calories you can consume per day, you should be choosing nutrient-rich foods over those that are nutrient poor. In doing so, you'll improve your chances of receiving an adequate amount of nutrients in your daily diet.

When you eat a processed food, you take in the same number of calories as a non-processed food, but fewer nutrients. These foods do a great job of filling your stomach, but a poor job of satisfying your hunger on a cellular level. So, even though you just had three meals today, your vital organs could still be lacking the nutrients they need. By choosing nutrient-dense foods, your nutrient intake will go up while the calorie count remains the same.

2. NUTRIENT DIVERSITY

In order for a food to be healthy, it needs to be nutrient dense across more than just one or two nutrients. Nutrient diversity simply means you are receiving a wide range of nutrients in a given period of time. The wider the spectrum of nutrients you receive, the higher the nutrient diversity.

There are two ways to add more nutrient diversity to your diet: (1) eat a wide variety of foods, or (2) select individual foods known for containing a variety of nutrients. No single food is perfect, so eating the same thing over and over will eventually lead to a nutrient deficiency—not to mention flavor boredom, right? Variety, after all, is the spice of life!

15,000 years ago, it was much easier to achieve nutrient diversity, as humans consumed an impressive 150 different ingredients per week. Over time, though, the availability of crop varieties has fallen. Just in the last century, over 75% of America's food diversity has disappeared. In 1903, for example, there were 497 varieties of lettuce available, but a mere 80 years later, there were just 36!

One reason for this stark drop in food diversity is because large, commercial farms began favoring crops able to grow in nutrient-poor soil, better withstand a harvest, ripen uniformly, and have longer shelf lives. Not only is this bad for nutrient diversity, but it also leads to crop failure, as insects and diseases have an easier time adapting to crop defenses when fewer varieties exist. Today, 90% of all calories consumed by humans worldwide come from a meager 14 animals and 30 crops. This trend and the risk it poses to the food supply in the future if one of these sources fails is troubling.

Another reason for the downward trend in crop varieties is due to human preference. Because we tend to prefer a certain flavor or food over another, the less favorable varieties eventually stop being produced. It's not hard to believe, then, that over 80% of convenience foods in America are made of just four ingredients: wheat, corn, soy, and meat.

Thankfully, there's still light at the end of the tunnel. Seed banks are working to preserve endangered crop varieties, and small, local farms continue to grow a wide variety of crops throughout the season. These farms typically select crops with high flavors and a variety of colors, favoring variation over uniformity and market preferences.

As a species, it's imperative that humans demand a greater variety of crops and reject convenience foods. This will send a message to commercial farms and food manufacturers and can make a significant difference not only to nutrient diversity for ourselves, but also to environmental sustainability for the entire planet.

3. NUTRIENT SYNERGY

"The whole is greater than the sum of its parts."

—*ARISTOTLE*

Nutrient synergy means nutrients found together in foods can have an amplification effect on each other, enhancing one another's beneficial properties or absorption into the body. As such, a food with a high amount of one nutrient but missing a complementary nutrient is nutritionally inferior to a food that contains adequate amounts of both nutrients.

We know that whole foods contain more vitamins, minerals, and phytonutrients than processed foods, but it's the potential synergistic effects between these nutrients that really sets them apart. Sweet potatoes, for example, have an abundance of nutrients like vitamin A, beta-carotene, vitamin C, vitamin B6, pantothenic acid, manganese, copper, iron, and fiber. But the synergies between these nutrients is what can further enhance the overall nutritional value of the food to an undetermined level.

There may be synergies between phytonutrients as well, which processed foods are lacking. One such phytonutrient group is flavonoids, which are linked to lower rates of diabetes and prostate cancer in men, and commonly found in whole foods like onions, apples, parsley, oranges, blueberries, bananas, bell peppers, and grapefruit.

Comparing foods doesn't have to be complicated. The next time you're faced with a difficult choice between two foods, make your assessment based on the three factors that allow you to determine which is the healthiest option: nutrient density, nutrient diversity, and nutrient synergy.

3

THE 37 MOST ESSENTIAL NUTRIENTS

"Separate the critical few from the trivial many."

—*TIM FERRISS*

Now that you've learned about the nutritional factors you need to measure when making a comparison between foods, it's time to discover which individual nutrients are most essential to life and everyday health. The 37 nutrients in this chapter were chosen because each is known to play a critical role in optimal health. Without them, your exposure to health-related risks and problems could increase.

In each nutrient section, you will find the following elements:

- an explanation of what the nutrient is and its benefits
- complications which may arise due to a deficiency
- the recommended daily intake
- any risks from consuming the nutrient in excess
- foods that are high in the nutrient

In my ranking analysis, which is explained in detail in the next chapter, only the first 34 nutrients were used. Nutrients 35, 36, and 37 were not included because either they do not currently exist in the USDA Nutritional Database, or there is not sufficient information available to make a recommendation. All 37 nutrients are important and essential, however, so be sure to include them as part of your daily diet or supplementation regimen.

1. VITAMIN K1

Vitamin K1, also known as phylloquinone, is important for healthy blood clotting and cardiovascular health. Specifically related to the heart, it is known to prevent and potentially reverse artery calcification caused by vitamin K deficiencies. Vitamin K1 is most abundantly found in green, leafy vegetables, like kale, collard greens, spinach, and parsley. The human body, however, is quite inefficient at absorbing this vitamin. At roughly 10% absorption, vitamin K1 is given less importance to its relative, vitamin K2, with a 100% absorption rate and nearly identical benefits.

Vitamin K1 deficiencies can lead to bleeding, osteoporosis, lowered life expectancy up to seven years,[3] and an underdeveloped face in deficiencies during infancy. Unwanted problems may occur if you consume inadequate or excessive amounts of vitamin K1. If you receive too little, you may experience bleeding of the gums, nose, and heavy menstrual bleeding in women, but too much and you may have difficulties with proper blood clotting, making you susceptible to excess bleeding in the event of a wound.

- Foodalytics Daily Intake (FDI) – 80 mcg [4]:182
- Upper Tolerance Level (UL), Toxicity – 10 mg/day [5]:257 This amount could be higher, as some studies indicate no adverse effects are associated with vitamin K intakes sourced from food or supplements.[6]

Foods high in vitamin K1 include kale, parsley, lambsquarters, spinach, mustard greens, collard greens, and beet greens.

2. VITAMIN K2

Vitamin K2, also known as menaquinone, has nine different subtypes: menaquinone-1 (MK-1) through menaquinone-9 (MK-9). Of all the subtypes, MK-4 and MK-7 are the most nutritionally important, but MK-8 and MK-9 are also commonly recognized. Nutritionally speaking, MK-4 has some benefits over MK-7, namely that it has a higher bioavailability (stays in the body longer and provides a longer-lasting effect). Nutritional values are available from the USDA for MK-4, so it will be the subtype referenced going forward and included in my nutritional scoring analysis.

In numerous studies, MK-4 has been found to be inversely related to severe aortic calcification and all-cause mortality,[7] as well as a reduction in bone loss and fractures.[8] Similar to vitamin K1, MK-4 plays an important role in proper blood clotting, as well as bone and cardiovascular health.[9] Vitamin K2 may also help treat and prevent certain cancers.[10]

MK-4 is commonly found in many fermented products, as well as meats. Kielbasa, a popular sausage in Poland, has between 13 and 17 mcg of MK-4 (depending on the cooking method used) and is 100% absorbable by the body. Kale, on the other hand, has a very high amount of K1, but at a 10% absorbable rate, the body only receives 10.62 mcg. Even though kale has more vitamin K2 (1062 mcg per serving), Kielbasa would be the healthier choice, as the total absorbancy is higher.

The recommended daily dosage of vitamin K2 varies widely. Some doctors recommend as little as 45 mcg/day, while researchers and academics recommend amounts as high as 500 to 2000 mcg/day.[11] Based on the majority of studies available, a daily dose of 600 mcg/day [4][12][13] seems to be the consensus and will be the recommendation given here.

- FDI – 600 mcg [4][12][13]
- UL, Toxicity – No adverse effects associated with vitamin K intake from food or supplementation.[6]

Foods high in vitamin K2 include chicken wings, chicken back, chicken thigh, chicken drumsticks, and chicken breast.

3. CHOLINE

Choline is important for methylation (building DNA, sending brain signals, liver detoxification), membrane structure production, and nervous system activity.

Signs and complications due to deficiencies include fatigue, Alzheimer's, memory loss, and cognitive and learning problems. According the National Health and Nutrition Examination Survey (NHANES) in 2003-2004, only 10% of Americans receive adequate amounts of choline in their diet.[14]

- FDI – 550 mg [15]
- UL, Toxicity – 3,500 mg [16]

Foods high in choline include egg yolk, whole egg, turkey breast, tri-tip roast, beef kidney, beef brain, and pork chitterlings.

4. FOLATE

Folate is a B vitamin that naturally occurs in food (not to be confused with folic acid, a synthetic form of vitamin B9, which many experts consider harmful to your health). A folate deficiency can cause severe birth defects, growth problems, and anemia.

- FDI – 400 mcg [15]
- UL, Toxicity – No UL from foods for adults.[17]:273[18] The UL for folate supplements or fortified foods is 1000 mcg.[16][17]:281[18] Folate UL for children and adolescents is 200 mcg for ages 1-3, 300 mcg for ages 4-5, 400 mcg for ages 7-10, 600 mcg for ages 11-14, and 800 mcg for 15-17.

Foods high in folate include chicken giblets, arrowroot, chickpea flour, cranberry beans, turkey liver, roasted soybeans, lentils, and edamame (frozen).

5. MANGANESE

Manganese is a trace mineral that helps promote strong bones, reduces the risk of osteoporosis, and is vitally important to the absorption of another essential nutrient, iron. It also plays a critical role in forming collagen in our skin, regulating blood sugar, and protecting the body from free radical damage.

- FDI – 2.3 mg [19]
- UL, Toxicity – 11 mg [5][20]

Foods high in manganese include beef liver, teff, rice bran, wheat germ, pine nuts, butternuts (dried), and wheat (hard red spring, hard red winter, or hard white).

6-7.OMEGA-3 (EPA AND DHA)

There are several strains of omega-3, but the following three are nutritionally the most significant: alpha-linolenic acid (ALA), eicosapentaenoic acid (EPA 20:5), and docosahexaenoic acid (DHA 22:6). EPA and DHA, in particular, are essential for producing vital cell membranes; at optimal levels, they may help prevent and treat several diseases. Complications due to an omega-3 deficiency may include rough or dry skin, acne, eczema, dull or dry hair, and soft or brittle nails.

The range of EPA and DHA recommendations vary from 217 mg to 1 gram per day for healthy adults. At the higher end, Chris Kresser, a popular health blogger and chiropractor, suggests individuals should consume roughly 1 gram per day to offset the high omega-6 intake in an average American diet. At high doses, omega-6 is said to cause inflammation in the body, which can lead to heart disease and other related conditions.[21]

With respect to general health and cardiovascular function, the National Institutes of Health (NIH) states that 650 mg of omega-3 fatty acids should be consumed per day. Of that amount, 217 mg should come from EPA and DHA.[22][23] In a medical paper released by the *American Journal of Clinical Nutrition* in 2006, the recommended amount for EPA and DHA was 500 mg per day. The paper noted that the "dietary strategy for achieving the 500-mg/d recommendation is to consume 2 fish meals per week (preferably fatty fish)."[24]

Similarly, the World Health Organization recommends between 300 to 500 mg of combined EPA and DHA per day,[25] which aligns well with biohacking pioneer Dave Asprey's suggestion that daily intakes should not exceed 350 mg for optimal brain function.[11]

There is no known toxic intake level for omega-3 from food sources. High levels of fish oil supplementation, on the other hand, could be problematic. In a 2010 study, patients receiving 3 grams of fish oil per day were observed to have increased LDL and insulin resistance.[26] Another study, however, saw the opposite results: statistically lower LDL, triglycerides, and improved oxidative stress markers.[27] While the evidence is mixed regarding fish oil supplementation, the safest bet would be to get your omega-3 by consuming fatty fish 1-2 times a week, as many of the concerns about the safety surrounding consuming whole fish have been unsubstantiated.

OMEGA-3 (EPA)

- FDI – 220 mg [23][24]
- UL, Toxicity – No limit.[5][28][29]

OMEGA-3 (DHA)

- FDI – 220 mg [23][24]
- UL, Toxicity – No limit.[5][28][29]

Foods high in omega-3 include salmon oil, mackerel, sockeye salmon, herring, sardine oil, wild-caught Atlantic salmon, menhaden oil, sardine oil, and wild caught Chinook salmon.

8. NIACIN (VITAMIN B3)

Niacin is important for energy production and antioxidant protection. Deficiencies can cause *pellagra*, with complications including diarrhea, dementia, skin problems, and even death. Excess niacin can cause flushing (a prickly heat sensation of the face and upper body).

- FDI – 16 mg [15]
- UL, Toxicity – 166 mg [5]

Foods high in B3 include turkey breast, rice bran, tri-tip roast (beef bottom sirloin), sockeye salmon, peanuts (Spanish, Virginia, or Valencia), chicken breast, and tuna (yellowfin).

9. THIAMINE (VITAMIN B1)

Thiamine is important for energy production and nervous system function. Deficiencies can lead to beriberi, a disease that can cause nerve, muscle, and heart damage, and may even affect the digestive system. Early warning signs of beriberi include shortness of breath, inflammation of the lower leg, and rapid heart rate during physical activity.

- FDI – 1.2 mg [15]
- UL, Toxicity – 500 mg [5]:96

Foods high in B1 include rice bran, spirulina, wheat germ, masa (corn flour), macadamia nuts, and tomatoes (canned).

10. VITAMIN B6

Vitamin B6 builds red blood cells and assists with liver detoxification and carbohydrate metabolism. It is important for optimum brain and nervous system function, but excess vitamin B6 can cause nerve problems. Although rare, complications due to a vitamin B6 deficiency include anemia and seizures.

- FDI – 1.3 mg [15]
- UL, Toxicity – 100 mg [20]

Foods high in vitamin B6 include turkey breast, rice bran, tri-tip roast (beef bottom sirloin), pistachios, garlic, wheat germ, and mamey sapote.

11. RIBOFLAVIN (VITAMIN B2)

Riboflavin (vitamin B2) is important for iron metabolism, energy production, and nervous system health. Deficiencies can cause ariboflavinosis, with complications as serious as coma and death.

- FDI – 1.3 mg [15]

- UL, Toxicity – None [17]:115

Foods high in riboflavin include lamb liver, spirulina, sweet whey, beef liver, beef kidney, pork heart, and pork kidney.

12. COPPER

Copper plays an important role in building strong bones and tissues and maintaining proper blood volume. It is a co-factor for one of the major antioxidant enzymes in the body called copper-zinc superoxide dismutase, which provides cells with a strong defensive barrier against oxygen toxicity and is a key player in maintaining a healthy immune system. Copper also plays an integral role in the synthesis of adenosine triphosphate (ATP), the body's primary energy source on a cellular level.

- FDI – 0.9 mg [19]
- UL, Toxicity – 10 mg [20]

Foods high in copper include lamb liver, spirulina, sesame seeds, beef sweetbread, beef liver, oysters, and breadnut tree seeds (dried).

13. VITAMIN D3

Vitamin D is critical for proper absorption of calcium in the bones. It is the #1 nutrient doctors recommend for supplementation due, in part, to recent spikes in cases of osteoporosis and rickets.

There are five different forms of vitamin D, of which two (D2 and D3) are especially important. In fact, the label "vitamin D" normally refers exclusively to these forms, unless otherwise specified. Vitamin D2 and D3 are fat soluble and chemically classified as secosteroids (steroids with a "broken" ring in their molecules).

Both forms of vitamin D are essential for calcium and phosphorus metabolism. Vitamin D2, which comes from plants and can be produced from ultraviolet light, aids in the production of insulin and helps the body fight tumors. Vitamin D3 comes from sunlight, and depending on the sun's angle, ten to twenty minutes is enough to provide what the body needs. Vitamin D3 aids in calcium absorption and retention, helps the immune system and the body regulate blood pressure, and helps prevent the following cancers: breast, colon, prostate, bladder, ovarian, and rectal.

When our skin is exposed to sunlight, a chemical process that produces vitamin D3 occurs in our bodies. "This D3, along with the D3 we get from food, gets converted by the liver into 25-hyrdroxy-vitamin D (25D), which is what typically gets measured when you have a vitamin D test. The optimal 25D level is somewhere between 35 and 50 ng/mL," states Chris Kresser, which is why he suggests daily vitamin D intakes of "somewhere between 2,000-5,000 IU."[30]

This falls in line with the Vitamin D Council daily dosage recommendation of 1000 IU for every 25 pounds of bodyweight for individuals.[31] In fact, they found that "taking 1000-4000 international units (IU) (25-100 mcg)/day of vitamin D may be associated with reduced pancreatic risk."[32]

As previously noted, a deficiency of vitamin D causes rickets, a disease in which the bones become so soft that they bend abnormally and can develop knobs. Children are commonly affected, developing unnatural poses such as knock-knees or bowed legs, which become permanent as the bones harden when they reach adulthood. Some studies show a link between a vitamin D deficiency and the development of Multiple Sclerosis (MS). Not surprisingly, recent research strongly suggests that MS sufferers whose diets are low in vitamin D are more likely to experience a relapse.

Suggestions regarding upper intake limits for vitamin D vary widely. The Vitamin D Council states there is no known upper limit for vitamin D3,[33] yet some studies found damaging effects at higher levels.[34] In fact, the Institute of Medicine (a component of the US National Academy of Sciences), states that "taking vitamin D supplements does not decrease risk of death, cardiovascular disease, or other conditions," which is why they recommend a more conservative range of 20 to 50 ng/mL.[35] Nevertheless, dosages of 50,000 IU and above are most associated with vitamin D toxicity symptoms.[36] Like many vitamins, D2 and D3 can be obtained in the form of supplements. D3, however, is much more prevalent.

- FDI – 125 mcg (5000 - 6000 IU)[31][32][30][11][37]
- UL, Toxicity - 1,000 to 1,250 mcg (40,000-50,000 IU)[36][38]

Foods high in vitamin D3 include halibut (raw), carp (raw), mackerel, eel (raw), sockeye salmon (canned), whitefish (smoked), and sockeye salmon.

14. IRON

Iron is important for the transportation of oxygen, which produces energy in the body. Iron deficiencies can cause anemia with symptoms including dizziness, lightheadedness, and fatigue.

- FDI – 8 mg [19]
- UL, Toxicity – 45-50 mg [5][20]

Foods high in iron include beef spleen, lamb spleen, beluga whale meat (dried), spirulina, rice bran, sesame seeds, and pork spleen.

15. MAGNESIUM

Magnesium is arguably one of the most important nutrients, alongside vitamin D. This vital nutrient acts on over 300 enzymes, aids in the strengthening of bones (reducing the risk of osteoporosis), improves blood circulation, and relaxes the nerves and muscles. Approximately 80% of Americans are, however, deficient in magnesium.

How can this be?

First, magnesium deficiencies often go undetected and untreated. It's difficult to detect a magnesium deficiency using a simple blood test, as the body is notoriously good at leaching magnesium from cells, bones, and tissues in order to maintain adequate blood levels of magnesium. Second, we're not getting as much magnesium from food sources as we did just 50-100 years ago. The earth's overall soil quality has decreased over time due to erosion and over-fertilization, thus magnesium levels passed from soil to food have been greatly reduced, making it difficult to get enough magnesium from food.[39]

Last, increased levels of stress, pharmaceutical drugs, and sugar intake all require magnesium and thus deplete stores in the body. For these reasons, many experts recommend daily magnesium supplementation.

Eating magnesium-rich foods is certainly another option, as well. Foods high in magnesium include rice bran, pumpkin and squash seeds, cottonseed, watermelon seeds (dried), soybean curd cheese, sesame seeds, and Brazil nuts. Eating approximately half a cup of pumpkin seeds will net you 382 mg of magnesium, bringing you close to the daily recommended amount for magnesium intake.

- FDI – 420 mg [19][30]
- UL, Toxicity – None [40]

16. CALCIUM

Calcium helps promote strong bones and reduces the risk of osteoporosis. Vitamin D and calcium often work together to build strong bones and having one without the other can become problematic. Parathyroid disorder, a disease in which the parathyroid gland is overactive, producing too much parathyroid hormone, can lead to a serious calcium imbalance. This is why Dr. Rakesh Patel advises patients to take calcium with vitamin D "to rule out potential parathyroid disorder masked by low [vitamin] D levels."

A calcium deficiency may lead to rickets. Calcium intake levels in excess of recommended dosages may prevent the absorption of iron and zinc in the body, cause constipation, and interfere with normal kidney function, which could lead to kidney stones.

- FDI – 1000 mg [19]
- UL, Toxicity – 2500 mg [5][20]

Foods high in calcium include sesame seeds, sisymbrium sp. seeds, swiss cheese, acid whey, whole milk (dried), sweet whey, and provolone cheese.

17. POTASSIUM

Potassium helps reduce blood pressure (which is why it's sometimes known as the anti-salt) and helps maintain a natural electrolyte balance. Excess potassium intake can cause hyperkalemia, which has no symptoms, but may lead to muscle weakness or dangerous heart rhythms.

- FDI – 4700 mg [19]
- UL, Toxicity – 4.7 g [19]

Foods high in potassium include radishes (dried), breadnut tree seeds (dried), sweet whey, turkey breast, roasted soybeans, cottonseed, and sun dried tomatoes.

18. ZINC

Zinc helps promote immune system function, eye health, taste function, male fertility, and skin health. A low level of zinc in the body is said to create a loss of taste or appetite. Signs of low zinc levels in the body include white spots on the fingernails.

- FDI – 11 mg [19]

- UL, Toxicity – 40-50 mg [5][20]

Foods high in zinc include oysters, tri-tip roast (beef bottom sirloin), beef chuck roast, chuck steak (boneless), top loin beef filet, beef ribeye filet, and wheat germ.

19. SELENIUM

Selenium is vital to maintaining normal thyroid function and plays a major role in supporting the antioxidant enzyme family, glutathione peroxidase (also known as selenoproteins). These antioxidants are crucial to the preservation of cell membranes and DNA integrity. Particularly, this enzyme family enhances glutathione's ability to react with free radicals, like hydrogen peroxide, turning these into harmless water molecules. If left untreated, hydrogen peroxide can break down further to become hydroxyl, an even more dangerous radical, which can damage cell membranes and DNA.

- FDI – 55 mcg [19]
- UL, Toxicity – 400 mcg [20] The UL for children and adolescents age 1-3 is 60 mcg, 4-6 is 90 mcg, 7-10 is 130 mcg, 11-14 is 200 mcg, and 15-17 is 250 mcg.[5]

Foods high in selenium include Brazil nuts, pork kidney, turkey breast, lamb kidney, wheat durum, tri-tip roast (beef bottom sirloin), and chicken giblets.

20. FIBER

Fiber is critical to digestive health. It is also important for maintaining a healthy colon and controlling blood sugar and cholesterol levels. There is no upper intake limit for fiber, as it is extremely difficult to over-consume this nutrient.

- FDI – 38 g [41]
- UL – None [42]

Foods high in fiber include corn bran (crude), carob flour, barley, chokecherries, rose hips, rye flour, and roasted soybeans.

21. PANTOTHENIC ACID (VITAMIN B5)

Pantothenic acid, also known as vitamin B5, supports the metabolism of fats and, like many B vitamins, plays an important role in energy production. A vitamin B5 deficiency can lead to paresthesia, which is associated with a pins and needles (tingling) feeling in the hands and feet, and can cause the limbs to fall asleep.

- FDI – 5 mg [15]
- UL, Toxicity – No limit.[5][16]

Foods high in vitamin B5 include sunflower seeds, turkey breast, rice bran, beef liver, sweet whey, chicken giblets, and egg yolk (dried).

22. PHOSPHORUS

Phosphorus is required for proper cell function, bone health, energy levels, and maintaining a good pH balance in the body. Deficiency risk of phosphorus is very low.

Some gastrointestinal issues were experienced in individuals with intakes of phosphorus exceeding 750 mg.[5] Other sources specify this level being upward of 4000 mg.[20]

- FDI – 700 mg [19]
- UL, Toxicity – 3000 mg [5]

Foods high in phosphorus include turkey breast, rice bran, pumpkin and squash seeds, sunflower seeds, sweet whey, and cottonseed.

23. VITAMIN A

Vitamin A plays a vital role in vision health and helps fight viruses in the body. A vitamin A deficiency is a leading cause of blindness in children and night blindness in adults. Excess vitamin A may lead to birth defects in infants.

With regard to upper tolerable intake levels, according to the American Society for Clinical Nutrition, "the safe upper single dose of retinol in oil or liver seems to be ~4-6 mg/kg body wt."[43] This means a 150-pound individual could consume up to 272,000 IU of vitamin A and still be safe. Furthermore, the risk of vitamin A toxicity is less pronounced in individuals who received adequate daily dosages of vitamin D3.[44]

While some may caution vitamin A intake recommendations for pregnant women, Chris Kresser commented at length on this topic, stating that the one study showing a correlation between vitamin A intake during pregnancy and toxicity has since been widely criticized and discredited. According to Kresser, "several other studies have not shown any increase in birth defects from vitamin A supplementation. On the contrary, most studies showed that mothers who supplemented with relatively high doses (10,000 IU) of vitamin A (even synthetic forms) had a lower risk of birth defects than mothers who didn't."[45]

- FDI – 10,000 IU (or 3,000 mcg of retinol)[43][30][11]
- UL, Toxicity – 272,000 IU (or 81,680 mcg of retinol)[43]

Foods high in vitamin A include beef liver, lamb liver, sweet potato, pumpkin (canned), butternut squash, carrots, and turkey liver.

24. VITAMIN C

Vitamin C boosts your immune system, is a natural antihistamine (which can provide relief for allergy symptoms such as nasal congestion, hives, and sneezing), and may help prevent and treat certain cancers. A vitamin C deficiency can lead to scurvy, a historically deadly disease common among sailors who did not have access to fresh fruits and vegetables during long voyages.

Possible complications from consuming excess vitamin C may include an increased risk of developing kidney stones.

Some sources point to an upper tolerable intake level of 2,000 mg for vitamin C, although others contend that extremely high doses are safe and effective at treating certain illnesses and diseases.

- FDI – 90 mg [46][15]
- UL, Toxicity – 2000 mg [5][16]

Foods high in vitamin C include acerola cherry, rose hips, guavas, yellow peppers, sweet red peppers, green peppers, and black currants.

25. VITAMIN E

Vitamin E protects against Alzheimer's and prostate cancer, reduces free radical damage, and offers UV protection. Complications due to deficiencies include muscle weakness and degeneration of the retina, which can cause blindness. Excess Vitamin E consumption may lead to hemorrhaging, a serious condition in which a ruptured blood vessel causes bleeding in the brain.[5][47]

- FDI – 15 mg [46][15][48]
- UL, Toxicity – 1000 mg [5][16]

Foods high in vitamin E include almonds, sunflower seeds, hazelnuts or filberts, granola, pine nuts, yellow pond lily seeds, and conch.

26. VITAMIN B12

Vitamin B12 has been shown to help prevent over 15 conditions: Alzheimer's, dementia, cognitive decline and memory loss, Multiple Sclerosis, mental illnesses (depression, anxiety, bipolar disorder, psychosis), cardiovascular disease, learning and developmental disorders in children, autism, autoimmune disease, cancer, and infertility.

A deficiency in vitamin B12 could increase your risk of developing hypocobalaminemia, a gradual deterioration of the spinal cord and/or brain, resulting in sensory or motor function loss, or any of the aforementioned conditions. Food sources of vitamin B12 are only found in animal products, which is why it's important for vegans and vegetarians to look to supplementation.

- FDI – 2.4 mcg [5][15]
- UL, Toxicity – No limit.[5][16]

Foods high in vitamin B12 include clams, beef liver, lamb kidney, lamb liver, octopus, beef kidney, and lamb brain.

27. BETA-CAROTENE

Beta-carotene helps prevent cancer, cardiovascular diseases like heart disease and stroke, and may lower the risk of contracting macular degeneration. Once ingested, beta-carotene is converted to retinol (vitamin A) and acts as an antioxidant, protecting cells from free radicals and oxidative damage.

Studies advise daily food intakes of beta-carotene between 3 to 6 mg in order to maintain beneficial blood level concentrations. These ranges have been shown to lower the risk of developing various chronic diseases. Epidemiological information linking high carotenoid intakes with lower cancer incidences dates back as far as the 1970s. The data suggests that patients with certain cancers (lung, oral, pharyngeal, and stomach) experienced the most protective effects. There was also a high correlation between alpha-carotene intake and a risk reduction of non-Hodgkin lymphoma.[49]

"Also noted was the apparent lack of toxicity of beta-carotene in high-dose clinical use against erythropoietic protoporphyria (doses of 20-300 mg/day given for many years)."[5]:19 A painful light sensitivity disorder, erythropoietic protoporphyria has been safely treated using therapeutic dosages of beta-carotene reaching levels of 180 mg/day.[48]:353,366

- FDI – 5000 mcg [48]:343,371
- UL, Toxicity – No limit [5][50][48]:366,371

Foods high in beta-carotene include sweet potato, pumpkin (canned), spinach, kale, carrots, mustard greens, and butternut squash.

28. ALPHA-CAROTENE

Similar to beta-carotene, alpha-carotene is also converted into retinol (vitamin A) and is referred to as a precursor to vitamin A. Alpha-carotene is known for its antioxidant properties, which protect the body against free radicals and oxidative damage. In particular, alpha-carotene helps prevent against lung[51] and other cancers, as well as cardiovascular disease (two of the leading causes of mortality). As expected, individuals with high serum levels of alpha-carotene are observed to have improved longevity.[52]

- FDI – 1500 mcg [48]:343
- UL, Toxicity – No limit.[48]:366

Foods high in alpha-carotene include pumpkin (canned), cooked pumpkin, raw pumpkin, raw carrots, butternut squash, and winter squash.

29. BETA-CRYPTOXANTHIN

Beta-cryptoxanthin is a member of the carotenoid family, which has been linked to reducing the risk of developing cancer, arthritis, oxidative damage, cognitive decline, diabetes, lung inflammation, obesity, and gum disease.

The National Center for Biotechnology Information (NCBI) ran a study that showed beta-cryptoxanthin intakes significantly decreased lung inflammation caused by cigarette smoking, with the greatest benefit coming from the high dose control group, which received 525 mcg per day. Specifically, "beta-cryptoxanthin has beneficial effects against cigarette smoke-induced lung inflammation, oxidative DNA damage, and lung squamous metaplasia and that beta-cryptoxanthin is a potentially effective chemopreventive agent against the development of lung cancer."[53][54] Similar findings were seen in the Singapore Health Study, in which a dosage of 550 mcg/day was associated with a significantly reduced risk of lung cancer.[55]

Blood level concentrations of 18 mcg/dL for beta-cryptoxanthin[48]:349 are associated with the lowest risk of age-related macular degeneration.

Individuals with low levels of both vitamin A and carotenoids (a precursor to vitamin A) are at risk of developing a vitamin A deficiency. Symptoms of a vitamin A deficiency include vision problems, dry skin, and an increased risk of infection.

- FDI – 525 mcg [53][54] up to 550 mcg [55]
- UL, Toxicity – No limit.[48]:366

Foods high in beta-cryptoxanthin include butternut squash, hubbard squash, persimmons, papayas, tangerines, and sweet red peppers.

30. LYCOPENE

Lycopene is a powerful antioxidant that plays a role in cancer prevention and is good for your eye and brain health. A member of the carotenoid family, lycopene helps reduce oxidative damage to DNA, which is one of the leading causes of heart disease.[56]

Long-term carotenoid deficiencies may increase the risk of tissue damage caused by free radicals.

Studies which administered lycopene to patients regarded 75 mg as the observed safe level, with much higher dosages resulting in no adverse effects.[57]

- FDI – 10 mg [58][59]
- UL, Toxicity – Likely no limit.[48]:366[60]

Foods high in lycopene include tomato sauce, sun-dried tomatoes, tomato juice, tomatoes (canned), rose hips, guavas, and cooked tomatoes.

31. LUTEIN+ZEAXANTHIN

Lutein+zeaxanthin is a carotenoid found in the human eye lens, retina, and macula. It is an antioxidant known to provide a significant benefit against the onset of adult-macular-degeneration (AMD) and cataracts. Low intakes of lutein+zeaxanthin could cause a deficiency in overall carotenoid levels, which may increase the risk of tissue damage caused by free radicals.

- FDI – 4.2 mg [48]:343[7]
- UL, Toxicity – No limit.[48]:366

Foods high in lutein+zeaxanthin include kale, spinach, swiss chard, mustard greens, turnip greens, collard greens, and garden cress.

32. FAT

Most research draws roughly the same conclusion: fats should fall somewhere between 20-35% of daily calories consumed.[61][62]:422 While modern experts recommend higher percentages ranging from 50 to 70%,[63][64] for the purposes of this book, a more conservative fat recommendation of 35% of energy needs was utilized.[65] Based on a 2,000 calorie diet, this translates to roughly 700 calories a day (or approximately 78 grams).

- FDI ~ 78 grams[65] with the following ratios: [66]
    - 40 g monounsaturated (52%)
    - 27 g saturated (35%)
    - 10 g polyunsaturated (13%)
    - 0 g trans fats (0%)
- UL, Toxicity – Not determined.[16][67]

Foods high in fat, by fat type:

- Monounsaturated fat – macadamia nuts, almonds, hazelnuts or filberts, pili nuts, pecans, hickory nuts, cashews.
- Saturated fat – coconut milk, pili nuts, beef fat, lamb fat, coconut meat (dried), heavy whipping cream.
- Polyunsaturated fat – butternuts, pine nuts, walnuts (black or white), sunflower seeds, watermelon seeds (dried).

33. PROTEIN

Protein is an important building block in the body for things like muscles, bones, hair and nails, skin, cartilage, and blood. A minimum of 0.8 grams of protein per kg of body weight is required for both men and women.[41]62]:645 A moderately higher ratio is recommended for the food rankings in the book, or approximately 1.4 grams per kg of body weight (98 grams/day for men and 80 grams/day for women), based on protein's beneficial role in healthy aging[76] and weight management.[77]

Maximum safe intake levels for protein range from 250 to 320 grams per day for a 70kg person (150 pounds).[68]

- FDI – 100 g [75][76][77]
- UL, Toxicity – 250-320 g [68]

Foods high in protein include turkey breast, tri-tip roast (beef bottom sirloin), roasted soybeans, sockeye salmon, spirulina, beef chuck roast, and cottonseed.

34. CARBOHYDRATES

According to the Institute of Medicine (US) and the Food and Nutrition Board, 130 g [41][62]:265 is the minimum brain requirement for carbohydrates. "This level of intake, however, is typically exceeded to meet energy needs while consuming acceptable intake levels of fat and protein."[62]:265 After accounting for fat and protein recommendations of 35 and 20 percent respectively, the remainder of energy needs is 45 percent for carbohydrates.

The the Institute of Medicine also suggests that a carbohydrate range of 45 to 65 percent is helpful for reducing the risk for CHD (coronary heart disease), obesity, and diabetes.[75] At this percentage, individuals should consume upward of 225 grams of carbohydrates per day to meet their caloric requirement.

For individuals that want to target lower carbohydrate intakes (for instance, 20 to 100 grams of carbs per day or less), they will need to increase their intake of fat or protein in order to safely meet their daily energy needs.

- FDI – 225 g [75]
- UL, Toxicity – Not determined.[16][67]

Foods high in carbohydrates include white rice, millet, teff, brown rice, triticale, sorghum, and wheat durum.

35. BIOTIN (VITAMIN B7)

Biotin helps the body maintain proper blood sugar levels and plays a role in skin health by forming fats in the skin cells. People who suffer from a biotin deficiency can develop skin rashes.

- FDI – 30 mcg [15]
- UL, Toxicity – Not Determined [16][67]

Foods high in biotin include almonds, sweet potato, eggs, onions, oats, and tomatoes.

36. IODINE

Iodine is vital for proper thyroid function, as well as skeletal and central nervous system development in infants.

Low end iodine recommendations start at 150 mcg per day,[19][69] moving up to doses of 325 mcg[70] and 1 mg per day.[11] At the high end of the spectrum, however, "physicians that specialize in treating hyperthyroidism with iodine... suggest doses as high as 50 mg per day."[70] For individuals without autoimmune disease, though, "a dose of 12.5 mg – 50 mg per day may be beneficial."[30]

- FDI – 12.5 mg [70]
- UL, Toxicity – 1,100 mcg [20]

Foods highest in iodine include sea vegetables (agar-agar, arame, dulse, kombu, nori, sea palm), scallops, cod, yogurt, shrimp, sardines, and salmon.[71]

37. FLAVONOIDS

Flavonoids are one of the largest phytonutrient groups, consisting of over 6,000 identified members that have been broken down into five major categories: flavonols, flavan-3-ols, flavones, flavanones, and anthocyanidins. Flavonoids are known for their antioxidant and anti-inflammatory properties, as well as their role in supporting the cardiovascular and nervous systems. They are also responsible for the deep reds in raspberries and deep blues in blueberries.

A decreased risk of lung and breast cancer is associated with flavonoid intakes, due to their role in the detoxification of molecules that can damage tissues. Similarly, flavonoids aid in the reduction of free radicals known to be harmful at the cellular level.

Quercetin, kaempferol, catechins, and anthocyanidins are some of the most well-known flavonoids. Since they are particularly sensitive to high heat, it's especially important to not use unnecessarily high temperatures when cooking foods containing flavonoids to preserve their nutrient content.

There is surprisingly little research information available with respect to flavonoids. As a result, flavonoid content could not be used in the food ranking analysis in this book.

- FDI – Unknown
- UL, Toxicity – Unknown

Foods high in flavonoids include onions, apples, parsley, oranges, blueberries, bananas, bell peppers, and grapefruit.

As you can see, there are many essential nutrients to keep be mindful of when you are making choices between foods. All 37 nutrients are important, and you need to make sure you receive adequate amounts of each of them. This is why I recommend paying attention to the *Foodalytics* rankings later in this book, as well as the Nutrition Facts in the Appendix, especially if there is a nutrient you need more of in your diet.

4

THE FOOD RANKING METHODOLOGY EXPLAINED

"The secret is there is no secret."

—*DAVE DRAPER*

When you eat healthier foods, your body receives more nutrients overall, significantly lowering your risk of developing one of 18 common nutrient deficiencies.[2] More nutrients means your chances of succumbing to one of these nutrient deficiencies—and their subsequent complications—is greatly reduced. Essentially, eating better foods means you're going to become healthier. It's that simple.

To calculate the food rankings listed in Part II of this book, I conducted a nutritional value analysis for over 8,900 foods (including various cooking types) using Release 28 of the USDA National Nutrient Database for Standard Reference. I computed an aggregate nutrient value for each food by totaling nutritional values across 37 essential nutrients with respect to the recommended Foodalytics Daily Intake (FDI) levels. I ranked the top 25 foods and then organized foods by food group, ranking the top 20 foods each.

Foodalytics Daily Intake (FDI)

Foodalytics Daily Intake (FDI) is a system of nutrient recommendations, derived from a variety of dietary intake references. It is the intake level that is considered sufficient for most healthy individuals for a given nutrient. FDI was a critical component of my analysis because it normalized the nutrient data, allowing me to combine unlike nutrients and compare one food's total nutrient value to another's.

For example, let's say Food A has 45 mcg of copper per serving and Food B has 45 mcg of zinc. At first, it would seem neither food is better than the other. If, however, you calculate the percent of daily requirement satisfied from each nutrient, and determine Food A provides 40% of your FDI for copper while

Food B provides only 15% of your FDI for zinc, we could safely conclude that Food A has more nutritional value per serving than Food B. Thus, Food A is healthier than Food B.

Nine of the essential nutrients did not have recommended amounts readily available, so suggested values were derived from medical research papers that recognized a health benefit at a specific intake level. Theses essential nutrients included vitamin K1, vitamin K2, omega-3 fatty acid (EPA and DHA), and the following phytonutrients: alpha-carotene, beta-carotene, beta-cryptoxanthin, lycopene, and lutein+zeaxanthin.

Tolerable Upper Intake Levels (UL)

I further normalized nutritional values using Tolerable Upper Intake Levels (UL). UL is the highest nutrient intake level likely to pose no risk of adverse health effects for most individuals.

So, for each nutrient, a UL cap was applied for two reasons: (1) to prevent foods from ranking higher due to extraordinarily high nutritional values per serving beyond the upper intake level (and therefore potentially unsafe) and (2) to allow foods that were nutritionally more well-rounded (having high nutrient diversity and nutrient synergy) to rank better.

For example, the UL level for selenium is 400 mcg per day. One serving of Brazil nuts, however, has approximately 2,549.6 mcg of selenium. In my nutrient scoring system, any amount over 400 mcg would not be counted, as no additional benefit would be derived from a value beyond the UL.

Food Groups Included

The following nine food groups were used to organize the top foods analyzed and ranked in this book:

1. Meat and Seafood
2. Vegetables
3. Fruits
4. Nuts and Seeds
5. Spices and Herbs
6. Dairy and Eggs
7. Legumes
8. Grains

9. Fats and Oils

Excluded Foods And Types

Processed foods, like sweets, restaurant foods, baby foods, fried foods, and beverages (including energy drinks, coconut water, and juices) were excluded. Raw meat was also excluded due to its potential health risks, as well as veal, due to the moral issues behind its consumption.

Cooking Preparation and Other Variables

The state in which foods are consumed is important to nutritional values. Each preparation method affects the nutritional properties for foods differently. Some nutrient values in foods are enhanced by a particular cooking method while others are diminished. The USDA nutrition facts were measured using various cooking methods for foods; for the most part, these properties were preserved in my ranking analysis food listings. Exceptions were made in certain cases, of course, as it's not feasible to consume things like raw legumes and most raw meats. The preparation methods included in this book are cooked, boiled, braised (dried) (canned), frozen, and even raw.

Sourcing of foods, as well as specific parts of foods, was also analyzed by the USDA. For example, turkey breast was measured both with and without the skin, and sockeye salmon was not only evaluated from a wild vs. farm caught perspective, but also with location as a consideration (the Atlantic vs. Pacific Ocean). This material was preserved, as well, in my data output, as it is important to know exactly why one food fared better than another. Although you might not have the luxury to import beef from New Zealand, you can remove the skin when baking your salmon or keep it on when cooking a chicken breast.

Other Food Ranking Systems

Ranking foods is not a new concept. For example, in 2014, the Centers for Disease Control and Prevention (CDC) produced a food report on the topic of superfoods. Four years prior to the superfoods report, however, Dr. Joel Fuhrman pioneered the popular food ranking system called ANDI, or Aggregate Nutrient Density Index. Whole Foods Market adopted the scoring system from 2010 to 2016 as part of their *Health Starts Here* campaign, which aimed to educate shoppers on how to make healthier food choices.

Below are some examples of ANDI scores from Dr. Fuhrman's website:

FOOD	ANDI SCORE
Kale	1000
Collard Greens	1000
Mustard Greens	1000
Watercress	1000
Salmon	34
Avocados	28
Olive Oil	9

The ANDI score is a system designed to rank foods based on nutrient density. The more nutrition per calorie, the higher the score. Despite its good intentions, there are some major shortcomings inherent to the ANDI ranking system.

First, the ANDI Score only lists 72 foods. This is because Dr. Fuhrman decided to only rank foods that are commonly eaten, rather than all foods. Foods like corn chips, vanilla ice cream, and cola made the list, but hundreds of common, healthy foods, like ginger, guavas, turkey, liver, thyme, Brazil nuts, quinoa, and oats were omitted.

Second, some foods scored surprisingly low on the index. While most would agree that kale likely deserves a top score of 1000, foods like avocados, olive oil, and salmon all received quite low scores, despite being widely regarded as some of the healthiest foods. For instance, salmon is in the top 1% in the Foodalytics rankings, yet placed in the bottom third under ANDI. Receiving a score of 34, that puts it behind corn and oatmeal and only marginally better than whole wheat bread.

Third, limiting yourself to the top foods in the ANDI system is dangerous, as many of the top foods provide few calories. This is because scores based on total nutrition per calorie, rather than per serving, and ignores daily caloric needs. Even if you wanted to, it would be virtually impossible to eat enough watercress to reach substantial energy levels. You could become starved very quickly, and if you fail to consider serving size long enough, you'd have no choice but to turn to potentially unhealthy foods to quickly fill the caloric void.

To explain why nutrient density works well in theory but not in practice, let's compare the biotin levels in both sweet potatoes and strawberries:

	Sweet Potato 1 cup, mashed (328 g)	**Strawberries** 1 cup, halves (152 g)
Biotin Per Serving	4.75 mcg	2.28 mcg
Biotin Per Calorie "Nutrient Density" (Biotin per 100 g / calories)	0.019	0.046
Calories	249	49

Source: Biotin levels from Staggs CG, Sealey WM, McCabe BJ, et al. Determination of the Biotin Content of Select Foods Using Accurate and Sensitive HPLC / Avidin Binding. J Food Compost Anal 2004;17:767-76.

If I asked you which food is better for biotin intake, and you subscribed to the nutrient density model, your answer would be strawberries because they have more than double the biotin per *calorie* than sweet potatoes (0.046 mcg versus 0.019 mcg). But if you followed the serving size model, you'd choose the sweet potato because you'd receive 4.75 mcg rather than 2.28 mcg of biotin per *serving*, which is more than double.

The biggest question here is, how much of a given food are you most likely to eat? I would argue that in most cases you are not going to always eat 100 grams of a food, and that you are most likely going to eat one serving. In this example, the ANDI system would require you to eat at least two servings of strawberries (that's 2 cups, which is quite a lot of berries) in order to match the biotin levels from just a single serving of sweet potatoes. While it's true that strawberries deliver more biotin per calorie consumed, it would be unlikely that you'd consume enough to receive more biotin than if you chose the sweet potato.

When it comes to making the best food choices each day, the *Foodalytics* rankings stand alone when compared to other food ranking systems. The number of foods ranked is comprehensive, all food groups are considered, and the recommendations are more applicable to your diet because they are founded upon practical serving sizes.

PART II

FOOD RANKINGS

5

THE TOP 25 HEALTHIEST FOODS

"Perfection is not attainable, but if we chase perfection
we can catch excellence."

—*VINCE LOMBARDI*

To recap what we've learned so far: we know what a nutrient is, what makes one food healthier than another, and the most essential nutrients necessary for everyday health. Now it's finally time to see the results. On the next page are the 25 healthiest foods. Each food has a calculated *Foodalytics* score next to it's name, based on total nutrients per serving.

Among the top 25:

- 12 are in the meat and seafood group
- 9 are vegetables (in case you didn't know, lambsquarters is a vegetable)
- 3 are in the nuts and seeds group
- 1 is in the grains group

Unfortunately, despite my crossed fingers, chocolate chip cookies didn't make the cut.

THE TOP 25 HEALTHIEST FOODS

RANK	FOOD	SCORE
1	Beef Liver	71.79
2	Lamb Liver	60.45
3	Clams	40.75
4	Turkey Breast	37.69
5	Lamb Kidney	37.24
6	Spinach (cooked or canned)	29.80
7	Kale	29.05
8	Sockeye Salmon	28.97
9	Rice Bran	28.91
10	Chicken Giblets	28.86
11	Sweet Potato	27.63
12	Pumpkin (canned)	27.03
13	Herring	26.74
14	Butternut Squash	25.69
15	Mackerel	24.75
16	Sesame Seeds	24.65
17	Seaweed, Spirulina (dried)	24.17
18	Mustard Greens	23.58
19	Lambsquarters	22.29
20	Tri-Tip Roast (Beef Bottom Sirloin)	22.26
21	Collard Greens	22.12
22	Sunflower Seed	21.88
23	Brazil Nuts	21.32
24	Oysters	20.86
25	Pork Liver	20.57

And there you have it: the top 25 healthiest foods! I know many of them are not what you might have expected, but I imagine a good number made sense. That's because much of what we know about healthy foods is either not based on fact, or is firmly rooted in conventional wisdom.

6

THE HEALTHIEST FOODS BY FOOD GROUP

"Knowing is not enough; we must apply.
Willing is not enough; we must do."
—*GOETHE*

This section of the book goes beyond just the top 25 healthiest foods and lists the top 20 foods for each of the nine food groups. As a reminder, those food groups are: meat and seafood, vegetables, fruits, nuts and seeds, spices and herbs, dairy and eggs, legumes, grains, and fats and oils.

Some of the top foods may surprise you, others you may have never heard of before, and the rest are common foods you can easily incorporate more into your daily meals.

#1. MEAT AND SEAFOOD

RANK	FOOD	SCORE
1	Beef Liver	71.79
2	Lamb Liver	60.45
3	Clams	40.75
4	Turkey Breast	37.69
5	Lamb Kidney	37.24
6	Sockeye Salmon	28.97
7	Chicken Giblets	28.86
8	Herring	26.74
9	Mackerel	24.75
10	Tri-Tip Roast (Beef Bottom Sirloin)	22.26
11	Oysters	20.86
12	Pork Liver	20.57
13	Pork Kidney	19.97
14	Sardines	19.80
15	Octopus	19.61
16	Turkey Liver	19.01
17	Turkey Giblets	18.69
18	Mussels	18.61
19	Beef Kidney	17.44
20	Lamb Brain	17.10

#2. VEGETABLES

RANK	FOOD	SCORE
1	Spinach (cooked or canned)	29.80
2	Kale	29.05
3	Sweet Potato	27.63
4	Pumpkin (canned)	27.03
5	Butternut Squash	25.69
6	Seaweed, Spirulina (dried)	24.17
7	Mustard Greens	23.58
8	Lambsquarters	22.29
9	Collard Greens	22.12
10	Swiss Chard	19.79
11	Beet Greens	17.82
12	Parsley	17.81
13	Turnip Greens	17.37
14	Dandelion Greens	14.97
15	Garden Cress	14.10
16	Carrots	13.77
17	Pokeberry Shoots	12.96
18	Pumpkin	12.61
19	Hubbard Squash	11.37
20	Radishes (dried)	10.44

#3. FRUITS

RANK	FOOD	SCORE
1	Acerola Cherry	19.03
2	Rose Hips	15.23
3	Peaches (dried)	7.98
4	Guavas	7.87
5	Persimmons	7.53
6	Mammy-Apple	7.38
7	Avocados	7.24
8	Prunes	5.99
9	Apricots (dried)	5.66
10	Passion-Fruit	5.49
11	Plums	5.08
12	Durian	5.02
13	Kiwi	4.58
14	Cantaloupe	4.49
15	Currants (dried)	4.44
16	Papayas	4.36
17	Pears (dried)	4.31
18	Sapote Mamey	4.06
19	Tangerines	3.99
20	Figs (dried)	3.98

#4. NUTS AND SEEDS

RANK	FOOD	SCORE
1	Sesame Seeds	24.65
2	Sunflower Seed	21.88
3	Brazil Nuts	21.32
4	Pine Nuts	19.72
5	Pumpkin and Squash Seeds	17.59
6	Cottonseed	17.16
7	Almonds	16.62
8	Butternuts (dried)	14.52
9	Walnuts, Black or White (dried)	14.40
10	Hazelnuts or Filberts	13.91
11	Cashews (dry roasted)	13.15
12	Pistachios	13.02
13	Breadnut Tree Seeds	12.28
14	Chestnuts	11.95
15	Hickory Nuts (dried)	11.83
16	Watermelon Seeds	11.11
17	Pecans	11.04
18	Macadamia Nuts	10.95
19	Pili Nuts	10.52
20	Coconut Milk	6.10

#5. SPICES AND HERBS

RANK	FOOD	SCORE
1	Paprika	1.24
2	Chili Powder	1.00
3	Cayenne or Red Pepper	0.85
4	Cloves (ground)	0.74
5	Turmeric (ground)	0.64
6	Thyme (dried)	0.52
7	Poppy Seed	0.45
8	Ginger (ground)	0.41
9	Cumin Seed	0.38
10	Cardamom	0.37
11	Fenugreek Seed	0.37
12	Celery Seed	0.37
13	Cinnamon (ground)	0.36
14	Basil (dried or fresh)	0.36
15	Curry Powder	0.33
16	Black Pepper	0.33
17	Mustard Seed (ground)	0.30
18	Coriander Leaf (dried)	0.29
19	Sage (ground)	0.29
20	Fennel	0.27

#6. DAIRY AND EGGS

RANK	FOOD	SCORE
1	Egg Yolk (dried)	14.99
2	Whole Egg (dried)	14.39
3	Sweet Whey	13.91
4	Whole Milk (dried)	11.04
5	Swiss Cheese	8.25
6	Feta Cheese	7.41
7	Cheddar Cheese	6.98
8	Acid Whey	6.86
9	Provolone Cheese	6.36
10	American Cheese Spread	6.30
11	Muenster Cheese	6.24
12	Colby Cheese	6.17
13	Brick Cheese	6.14
14	Limburger Cheese	6.08
15	Monterey Cheese	6.02
16	Fontina Cheese	5.98
17	Port De Salut Cheese	5.81
18	Parmesan Cheese	5.73
19	Hard Boiled Egg	5.68
20	Mexican Cheese (queso anejo)	5.62

#7. LEGUMES

RANK	FOOD	SCORE
1	Peanuts (Spanish, Virginia, Valencia)	14.94
2	Soybeans (roasted)	13.89
3	Soy Flour (full-fat, roasted)	10.55
4	Natto	10.37
5	Soybean Curd Cheese	9.59
6	Tempeh	6.74
7	Chickpea Flour (Besan)	6.72
8	Winged Beans	6.12
9	Lentils	5.96
10	Adzuki Beans	5.87
11	White Beans	5.71
12	Navy Beans	5.61
13	Great Northern Beans	5.60
14	Chickpeas	5.53
15	Baked Beans	5.07
16	Pink Beans	5.01
17	Pinto Beans	4.97
18	Hyacinth Beans	4.91
19	Yellow Beans	4.88
20	Small White Beans	4.84

#8. GRAINS

RANK	FOOD	SCORE
1	Rice Bran	28.91
2	Wheat Germ	18.88
3	Teff	15.91
4	Amaranth Grain	14.93
5	Wheat Durum	14.63
6	Wheat (Hard Red Spring, Hard Red Winter, or Hard White)	14.52
7	Quinoa	11.94
8	Oats	11.69
9	Rye Flour	11.47
10	Granola	11.36
11	Barley (hulled)	11.33
12	Spelt	10.95
13	Millet	10.65
14	Wheat (Soft Red Winter or Soft White)	10.52
15	Triticale	9.95
16	Brown Rice (long grain)	9.87
17	Buckwheat	9.86
18	Rye Grain	9.67
19	Oat Bran	9.11
20	Brown Rice Flour	9.10

#9. FATS AND OILS

RANK	FOOD	SCORE
1	Salmon Oil	20.07
2	Menhaden Oil	14.14
3	Sardine Oil	13.55
4	Herring Oil	6.99
5	Cod Liver Oil	5.35
6	Safflower Oil (linoleic, over 70%)	1.42
7	Grapeseed Oil	1.32
8	Cottonseed Oil	1.26
9	Poppyseed Oil	1.09
10	Flaxseed Oil (cold pressed)	1.05
11	Rice Bran Oil	1.05
12	Walnut Oil	1.01
13	Oat Oil	0.95
14	Canola Oil	0.94
15	Tomatoseed Oil	0.93
16	Almond Oil	0.88
17	Hazelnut Oil	0.87
18	Peanut Oil	0.82
19	Sesame Oil	0.81
20	Wheat Germ Oil	0.79

7

SEVEN MYTHS ABOUT THE HEALTHIEST FOODS: BUSTED

"The great enemy of the truth is very often not the lies, deliberate, contrived and dishonest, but the myth, persistent, persuasive and unrealistic."

—*JOHN F. KENNEDY*

Reflecting on the healthiest food rankings in *Foodalytics*, many of our previously held beliefs hold true, but there are still some surprising results. Foods once thought to hold a top position as a healthy food have been outranked, while others are missing entirely.

Using nutritional information, we are able to question these assumptions and take a factual stance. I'd like to take this opportunity to dispel the seven biggest myths I see regarding the healthiest foods.

SEVEN MYTHS ABOUT THE HEALTHIEST FOODS

1. **Kale and spinach are the healthiest foods.** Contrary to popular belief, these foods are not even in the top 5, with spinach at #7 and kale at #8. Beef and lamb liver beat out these foods, with beef liver containing more than double the nutritional intake of either spinach or kale.

2. **Meat, other than fatty fish like salmon, isn't healthy for you.** Salmon is well-positioned at #9, but the high rankings of organ meats and turkey breast prove that meat really has more to offer, as far as nutrition is concerned. A number of other seafood options also made the cut, like clams, herring, mackerel, and oysters.

3. **Liver is bad for you because it is full of toxins.** Among health experts, liver is widely accepted as one of nature's healthiest foods. Contrary to popular belief, liver is not full of toxins. In fact, the liver's job is to *neutralize* toxins, not store them. The liver stores important nutrients such as vitamin A, D, E, K, B12, folic acid, copper and iron, which actually help the body *remove* toxins.[72] Liver really is the most nutritionally rich and healthiest food on Earth!

4. **Fruits and vegetables are the healthiest food groups.** Wrong! While it is important to eat fruits and greens for the nutrients, fiber, and phytonutrients they contain, the meat and seafood food group commands the throne. Fruits occupy 0% of the top 25 foods, grains are at 4%, nuts and seeds 12%, vegetables 36%, and meat and seafood take the crown at 48%.

5. **Grains offer very little nutritional value.** This isn't necessarily true. While only one grain made the top 25 foods, rice bran managed to land very high on the list at #10. I'll talk more about rice bran in Chapter 8, but it is packed with a wide variety of nutrients.

6. **Nuts and seeds are fatty and not very nutrient-dense or well-rounded.** Nuts and seeds deserve our attention, as they make up a cool 12% of the healthiest foods in the top 25. With three distinct foods joining the ranks (sesame seeds, sunflower seeds, and Brazil nuts), we would be wise to include more of them in our regular diets.

7. **Dark, leafy greens are the only vegetables worth eating.** This is definitely untrue! Many of the non-green vegetables that made the top 25 did so because they contain high amounts of carotenoids, a very healthy phytonutrient group known to help prevent deadly diseases like cancer, as well as a plethora of other essential nutrients. The three non-green veggies that made the grade are sweet potato, pumpkin (canned), and butternut squash.

Understanding the truth behind a myth is necessary for us to be able to move past these limiting beliefs and start making healthy food choices. The sooner we do this, the sooner we can begin strengthening our bodies to better fend off disease, improve function, and expand longevity.

8

HOW TO INCORPORATE THE HEALTHIEST FOODS INTO YOUR DIET

"There is not one path.
There is not even the right path.
There is only your path."
—*SUE KREBS*

Awareness of the healthiest foods is a great start, but if you really want to set yourself up for success, you're going to need to know how to incorporate them into your daily meal plans. As you know, in the top 25 we have 12 meat and seafood foods, 9 vegetables, 3 nuts and seeds, and 1 grain. A typical day could include one to two items from the meat and seafood group, one item from the vegetable group, and an optional nut and seed selection. Finally, once a week you can incorporate rice bran, the sole grain to make the cut.

Let's break down each of the food groups further, into specific examples of foods you could choose in a given day or week, to ensure you experience as many of the healthiest foods as possible.

MEAT AND SEAFOOD

Within the meat and seafood group, 5 are seafood (clams, salmon, herring, mackerel, and oysters), 5 are organ meats (beef liver, lamb liver, lamb kidney, chicken giblets, and pork liver), and the remaining 2 are turkey breast and beef roast.

The biggest takeaway here is to try to incorporate more organ meats and seafood items into your weekly meals. The easiest organ meat to find is beef liver, as just about every local grocery store carries it. Kidney and giblets will be harder to come by, but you can start at your local butcher shop or farm. If there aren't any shops like this around you, buying online is another option. Places like US Wellness Meats (grasslandbeef.com) will ship frozen meats directly to your door overnight.

The best way to add more organ meats to your diet is to start small. If you can choose one organ meat per week, that would be fantastic, but every other week or once a month might be where the majority of you will start. By themselves, organ meats can taste bland, so cooking them with seasoning, along with other flavorful foods (onions, garlic, bacon, etc.) can really be the difference between never eating them and having them regularly.

As for other meals during the week, you should have no problem getting your hands on turkey breast, beef roast, or any of the healthy seafood options (clams, herring, mackerel, and oysters).

VEGETABLES

If you plan to eat approximately one vegetable per day, you can just about fit in all the recommended vegetables in a given week. The nine vegetables that made the list fall into two main categories: greens and starchy vegetables.

To further break down the greens, four are dark, leafy greens (spinach, kale, mustard greens, and collard greens) and the other two are more unconventional: lambsquarters and spirulina. A lighter-colored green leaf, lambsquarters is considered by some to be a weed, but it can be used in salads or cooked and added to a variety of dishes similar to how you would use spinach. Spirulina is essentially algae and isn't feasible to obtain or consume in its natural state but is available in powdered and tablet form. Spirulina can easily be sprinkled into drinks and smoothies, directly onto solid foods, or added to your daily supplementation regime.

Starchy vegetables in the top 25 food rankings include sweet potato, pumpkin (canned), and butternut squash. These foods have made their way into many US households, but most likely on a less-than-regular basis. If you would like to consume one of each starchy vegetable per week, aim to eat one every other day.

NUTS AND SEEDS

Nuts and seeds are a great snack food or garnish. The following nuts and seeds made the top cut: sesame seeds, sunflower seeds, and Brazil nuts.

Easy ways to add them to your daily meals would be to sprinkle them on a salad, or buy a bag of them to snack on (sesame seeds are too small to consume or manufacture for snack purposes, unfortunately). These bagged snacks can be eaten in the office, on the go, or at home.

There are a number of recipes that call for grinding or pulverizing Brazil nuts, after which they can be added to just about anything. You can even create your own healthy, butter-like spread!

GRAINS

Rice bran is the outer shell on a grain of rice. Until the 90s, no one knew how to separate the bran and germ from the rice kernel without damaging their fragile nutrition. Usually discarded after processing white rice, rice bran is a highly nutritious, well-rounded food. It comes in the same form as many grains and can be easily added to smoothies or baked goods.

When you break down the top 25 foods into smaller parts, it's plain to see which foods can easily be incorporated into our weekly meal plans and which will take a little more effort. The good news is you really can't go wrong here, because every effort you make to include more of these foods in your diet is a step toward better health. Plus—who knows?—you might fall in love with some of these nutrient-packed foods and get others to do the same!

FOODALYTICS RECIPES

For even more ways to incorporate the healthiest foods into your diet, head on over to http://FoodalyticsBook.com/Recipes to find some delicious meals you can try out today.

9

THE IMPORTANCE OF BALANCE

"Balance is the key to success in all things."

—TANYA WHEWAY

No doubt, a listing of the top 25 healthiest foods is your ultimate resource as you continue along your health journey. But a word of caution: choosing the same foods repeatedly is a recipe for disaster, as no single food has the perfect assortment of nutrients. To ensure that you safely bringing your health to the next level, you should strive for moderation in your diet.

Eating a variety of foods across all of the food groups is one of the best ways to achieve this healthy balance. Where one food may be weak in some nutrients, others will be strong. By frequently choosing new foods and food groups, you will greatly reduce your chances of suffering from a nutrient deficiency.

Another strategy you can use is to consume fresh fruits and vegetables that are in season. Not only does this ensure you're eating a wide variety of foods, but it also further optimizes your nutritional intake. This is because eating fruits and vegetables shortly after they are grown minimizes the time they have to decay and maximizes the total nutrient content received. The moment foods are harvested or picked, they begin to ripen and lose color, flavor, and nutrients.

Some situations may require more or less of a particular nutrient. If you are not supplementing with vitamin A, organ meats should be eaten twice a week or more. Consuming organ meats every day could be problematic, as the over-consumption of certain vitamins and minerals could lead to toxicity. Similarly, fruits containing high amounts of fructose (a natural fruit sugar) should be eaten in limited quantities.

No matter what diet you subscribe to, you should ensure you're receiving an adequate nutrient intake for each of the essential vitamins and minerals listed in Chapter 3. If you eliminate a food group from your diet, it is important that you understand which nutrients you will be low in and look to supplementation in order to get your nutrient intake to the recommended levels.

CONCLUSION

When we eat better, we become healthier. For the majority of you, armed with this information, there's a lot you can do to improve the nutritional quality of the food you eat. For those of you who have eaten healthy for a number of years, there are small tweaks you can make, like swapping out a less nutritious food for one that's more nutritious, to take your health to the next level.

By now, you know food is not just something to consume for pleasure, but a vehicle in which nutrients are the passenger. The 37 most essential nutrients are the building blocks for creating and repairing cells, provide your body with a primary source of energy, and are a catalyst for achieving optimal human performance.

With *Foodalytics*, you now have the information you need to attain your health and nutritional goals. If you continue to take action and choose quality foods, I'm confident you will be able to maximize your nutrient intake and live a long and healthy life.

Remember to always have fun, try new foods, and above all: enjoy your newfound health and vitality!

WOULD YOU DO ME A FAVOR?

Before you go, I'd like to thank you for purchasing my book. You could have picked dozens of different books on health, but you took a chance with mine, so thanks for choosing this book and reading all the way to the end.

If you liked what you read, I could use your help!

Please take a moment to leave a review for this book on Amazon:

http://FoodalyticsBook/Review

This feedback will help me continue to write books for improving your health. If you loved this one, please let me know! :-)

PART III

APPENDIX AND REFERENCES

APPENDIX: HEALTHIEST FOODS NUTRITION FACTS

The remainder of the book provides nutrition facts calculated for each of the healthiest foods, including the scoring and ranking figures that were essential to conducting the analysis.

Summary of the Nutrition Facts:

- Each nutrition fact is for one food and one serving.
- FDI stands for Foodalytics Daily Intake. This is the recommended amount of a given nutrient a healthy adult should aim to receive each day.
- UL stands for Tolerance Upper Intake Level. The UL is the point at which a given nutrient value is no longer beneficial to the body. Rather, it has surpassed a toxicity threshold.
- Any FDI percentage over and above the UL was not counted for the rankings. However, in the rankings the full percentage was included.

All nutrition facts for each of the foods were calculated using Release 28 of the USDA National Nutrient Database for Standard Reference.[73]

MEAT AND SEAFOOD

Nutrients per One Serving

#1 Beef Liver

Total Nutrient Score of 71.79
Overall Rank: 1 of 8990
Meat and Seafood Rank: 1 of 20
Serving Size: 3 oz (85 g)
Cooking preparation(s): cooked, boiled
Calories: 128 | Carbs: 3.21 g

12122% FDI for Manganese *UL used for ranking analysis
3400% FDI for Vitamin B12
1985% FDI for Vitamin A
541% FDI for Copper
199% FDI for Riboflavin (Vitamin B2)
167% FDI for Pantothenic Acid (Vitamin B5)
76% FDI for Iron
73% FDI for Niacin (Vitamin B3)
48% FDI for Phosphorus
40% FDI for Omega-3 (EPA, 20:5)
30% FDI for Vitamin B6
27% FDI for Thiamine (Vitamin B1)
26% FDI for Zinc
25% FDI for Selenium
20% FDI for Protein
14% FDI for Omega-3 (DHA, 22:6)
7% FDI for Vitamin E
7% FDI for Fats - Polyunsaturated
6% FDI for Potassium
4% FDI for Fats - Saturated
4% FDI for Magnesium
1% FDI for Carbohydrate
1% FDI for Fats - Monounsaturated

#2 Lamb Liver

Total Nutrient Score: 60.45
Overall Rank: 2 of 8990
Meat and Seafood Rank: 2 of 20
Serving Size: 3 oz (85 g)
Cooking preparation: cooked, soaked and fried
Calories: 143 | Carbs: 1.26 g

2037% FDI for Vitamin B12
1877% FDI for Vitamin A
1266% FDI for Copper *UL used for ranking analysis
345% FDI for Riboflavin (Vitamin B2)
111% FDI for Thiamine (Vitamin B1)
89% FDI for Pantothenic Acid (Vitamin B5)
80% FDI for Omega-3 (DHA, 22:6)
68% FDI for Niacin (Vitamin B3)
63% FDI for Omega-3 (EPA, 20:5)
57% FDI for Iron
56% FDI for Phosphorus
39% FDI for Zinc
29% FDI for Selenium
22% FDI for Protein
14% FDI for Manganese
12% FDI for Vitamin B6
10% FDI for Fats - Polyunsaturated
6% FDI for Vitamin E
6% FDI for Fats - Saturated
5% FDI for Potassium
4% FDI for Magnesium
2% FDI for Fats - Monounsaturated

#3 Clams

Total Nutrient Score: 40.75
Overall Rank: 3 of 8990
Meat and Seafood Rank: 3 of 20
Serving Size: 3 oz (85 g)
Cooking preparation: cooked, moist heat
Calories: 126 | Carbs: 4.36 g

3503% FDI for Vitamin B12
99% FDI for Selenium
65% FDI for Copper
56% FDI for Omega-3 (DHA, 22:6)
53% FDI for Omega-3 (EPA, 20:5)
41% FDI for Phosphorus
37% FDI for Manganese
30% FDI for Iron
28% FDI for Riboflavin (Vitamin B2)
22% FDI for Protein
21% FDI for Zinc
21% FDI for Vitamin C
18% FDI for Niacin (Vitamin B3)
16% FDI for Vitamin A
12% FDI for Pantothenic Acid (Vitamin B5)
11% FDI for Potassium
11% FDI for Thiamine (Vitamin B1)
8% FDI for Calcium
7% FDI for Vitamin B6
6% FDI for Folate
5% FDI for Fats - Polyunsaturated
4% FDI for Magnesium
2% FDI for Carbohydrate

#4 Turkey Breast (meat only)

Total Nutrient Score: 37.69
Overall Rank: 4 of 8990
Meat and Seafood Rank: 4 of 20
Serving Size: 1 breast (863 g)
Cooking preparation: cooked, roasted
Calories: 1174 | Carbs: 0 g

634% FDI for Niacin (Vitamin B3)
633% FDI for Vitamin B12
551% FDI for Vitamin B6
482% FDI for Selenium
312% FDI for Phosphorus
255% FDI for Protein *UL used for ranking analysis
179% FDI for Pantothenic Acid (Vitamin B5)
126% FDI for Riboflavin (Vitamin B2)
120% FDI for Choline
119% FDI for Zinc
105% FDI for Iron
58% FDI for Fats - Polyunsaturated
58% FDI for Magnesium
58% FDI for Copper
55% FDI for Potassium
31% FDI for Thiamine (Vitamin B1)
21% FDI for Fats - Saturated
20% FDI for Omega-3 (DHA, 22:6)
20% FDI for Folate
14% FDI for Fats - Monounsaturated
12% FDI for Calcium
4% FDI for Omega-3 (EPA, 20:5)
3% FDI for Vitamin E
3% FDI for Vitamin A
2% FDI for Manganese
1% FDI for Lutein+Zeaxanthin
1% FDI for Vitamin D3

#5 Lamb Kidney

Total Nutrient Score: 37.24
Overall Rank: 5 of 8990
Meat and Seafood Rank: 5 of 20
Serving Size: 3 oz (85 g)
Cooking preparation: cooked, braised
Calories: 116 | Carbs: 0.84 g

2795% FDI for Vitamin B12
338% FDI for Selenium
135% FDI for Riboflavin (Vitamin B2)
132% FDI for Iron
35% FDI for Phosphorus
35% FDI for Copper
35% FDI for Pantothenic Acid (Vitamin B5)
32% FDI for Niacin (Vitamin B3)
29% FDI for Zinc
25% FDI for Thiamine (Vitamin B1)
23% FDI for Omega-3 (EPA, 20:5)
20% FDI for Protein
17% FDI for Folate
15% FDI for Omega-3 (DHA, 22:6)
13% FDI for Vitamin A
11% FDI for Vitamin C
8% FDI for Vitamin B6
6% FDI for Fats - Polyunsaturated
5% FDI for Manganese
4% FDI for Magnesium
4% FDI for Fats - Saturated
3% FDI for Potassium
2% FDI for Fats - Monounsaturated
2% FDI for Calcium

#6 Sockeye Salmon

Total Nutrient Score: 28.97
Overall Rank: 7 of 8990
Meat and Seafood Rank: 6 of 20
Serving Size: 1 filet (108 g)
Cooking preparation: filets with skin, smoked
Calories: 373 | Carbs: 0 g

815% FDI for Vitamin B12
746% FDI for Omega-3 (DHA, 22:6)
444% FDI for Omega-3 (EPA, 20:5)
154% FDI for Niacin (Vitamin B3)
149% FDI for Selenium
100% FDI for Phosphorus
68% FDI for Vitamin B6
65% FDI for Protein
59% FDI for Pantothenic Acid (Vitamin B5)
45% FDI for Riboflavin (Vitamin B2)
45% FDI for Thiamine (Vitamin B1)
44% FDI for Choline
37% FDI for Fats - Polyunsaturated
22% FDI for Potassium
18% FDI for Copper
15% FDI for Magnesium
14% FDI for Iron
11% FDI for Zinc
11% FDI for Fats - Monounsaturated
10% FDI for Fats - Saturated
9% FDI for Vitamin E
6% FDI for Calcium
4% FDI for Vitamin A
3% FDI for Folate
2% FDI for Manganese

#7 Chicken Giblets

Total Nutrient Score: 28.86
Overall Rank: 8 of 8990
Meat and Seafood Rank: 7 of 20
Serving Size: 1 cup, chopped or diced (145 g)
Cooking preparation: cooked, fried
Calories: 402 | Carbs: 6.31 g

804% FDI for Vitamin B12
577% FDI for Vitamin A
275% FDI for Selenium
187% FDI for Iron
170% FDI for Riboflavin (Vitamin B2)
138% FDI for Folate
129% FDI for Pantothenic Acid (Vitamin B5)
100% FDI for Niacin (Vitamin B3)
83% FDI for Zinc
68% FDI for Vitamin B6
68% FDI for Copper
59% FDI for Phosphorus
49% FDI for Fats - Polyunsaturated
47% FDI for Protein
26% FDI for Omega-3 (DHA, 22:6)
20% FDI for Fats - Saturated
16% FDI for Fats - Monounsaturated
14% FDI for Manganese
14% FDI for Vitamin C
12% FDI for Thiamine (Vitamin B1)
10% FDI for Potassium
9% FDI for Magnesium
6% FDI for Omega-3 (EPA, 20:5)
3% FDI for Carbohydrate
3% FDI for Calcium

#8 Herring

Total Nutrient Score: 26.74
Overall Rank: 13 of 8990
Meat and Seafood Rank: 8 of 20
Serving Size: 1 fillet (143 g)
Cooking preparation: cooked, dry heat
Calories: 290 | Carbs: 0 g

783% FDI for Vitamin B12
718% FDI for Omega-3 (DHA, 22:6)
591% FDI for Omega-3 (EPA, 20:5)
122% FDI for Selenium
62% FDI for Phosphorus
39% FDI for Fats - Polyunsaturated
38% FDI for Vitamin B6
37% FDI for Niacin (Vitamin B3)
33% FDI for Protein
33% FDI for Riboflavin (Vitamin B2)
25% FDI for Iron
22% FDI for Choline
21% FDI for Pantothenic Acid (Vitamin B5)
19% FDI for Copper
17% FDI for Fats - Monounsaturated
17% FDI for Zinc
14% FDI for Magnesium
14% FDI for Fats - Saturated
13% FDI for Thiamine (Vitamin B1)
13% FDI for Vitamin E
13% FDI for Potassium
11% FDI for Calcium
6% FDI for Vitamin D3
6% FDI for Vitamin A
4% FDI for Folate
2% FDI for Manganese
1% FDI for Vitamin C

#9 Mackerel

Total Nutrient Score: 24.75
Overall Rank: 15 of 8990
Meat and Seafood Rank: 9 of 20
Serving Size: 1 piece (5-1/2" x 1-1/2" x 1/2") (80 g)
Cooking preparation: salted
Calories: 244 | Carbs: 0 g

1078% FDI for Omega-3 (DHA, 22:6)
589% FDI for Omega-3 (EPA, 20:5)
400% FDI for Vitamin B12
107% FDI for Selenium
50% FDI for Fats - Polyunsaturated
29% FDI for Phosphorus
25% FDI for Vitamin B6
21% FDI for Fats - Saturated
17% FDI for Fats - Monounsaturated
17% FDI for Niacin (Vitamin B3)
16% FDI for Vitamin D3
15% FDI for Protein
15% FDI for Choline
14% FDI for Iron
13% FDI for Vitamin E
12% FDI for Riboflavin (Vitamin B2)
11% FDI for Magnesium
9% FDI for Copper
9% FDI for Potassium
8% FDI for Zinc
8% FDI for Vitamin K1
5% FDI for Calcium
4% FDI for Vitamin A
3% FDI for Folate
1% FDI for Thiamine (Vitamin B1)

#10 Tri-Tip Roast (Beef Bottom Sirloin)

Total Nutrient Score: 22.26
Overall Rank: 20 of 8990
Meat and Seafood Rank: 10 of 20
Serving Size: 1 roast (yield from 690 g raw meat) (569 g)
Cooking preparation: cooked, roasted
Calories: 1201 | Carbs: 0 g

363% FDI for Vitamin B12
290% FDI for Selenium
247% FDI for Niacin (Vitamin B3)
242% FDI for Zinc
239% FDI for Vitamin B6
163% FDI for Phosphorus
148% FDI for Protein
118% FDI for Iron
103% FDI for Choline
59% FDI for Pantothenic Acid (Vitamin B5)
55% FDI for Riboflavin (Vitamin B2)
49% FDI for Copper
39% FDI for Potassium
33% FDI for Thiamine (Vitamin B1)
30% FDI for Magnesium
15% FDI for Vitamin E
12% FDI for Folate
11% FDI for Calcium
10% FDI for Vitamin K1
2% FDI for Manganese

#11 Oysters

Total Nutrient Score: 20.86
Overall Rank: 24 of 8990
Meat and Seafood Rank: 11 of 20
Serving Size: 3 oz (85 g)
Cooking preparation: cooked, moist heat
Calories: 87 | Carbs: 4.63 g

620% FDI for Vitamin B12
607% FDI for Zinc *UL used for ranking analysis
539% FDI for Copper
136% FDI for Omega-3 (EPA, 20:5)
105% FDI for Omega-3 (DHA, 22:6)
98% FDI for Iron
61% FDI for Selenium
24% FDI for Phosphorus
22% FDI for Manganese
20% FDI for Choline
12% FDI for Riboflavin (Vitamin B2)
10% FDI for Calcium
10% FDI for Niacin (Vitamin B3)
10% FDI for Protein
10% FDI for Vitamin E
9% FDI for Fats - Polyunsaturated
8% FDI for Pantothenic Acid (Vitamin B5)
7% FDI for Magnesium
4% FDI for Vitamin B6
3% FDI for Folate
3% FDI for Fats - Saturated
3% FDI for Thiamine (Vitamin B1)
3% FDI for Potassium
3% FDI for Vitamin A
2% FDI for Vitamin K1
2% FDI for Carbohydrate
1% FDI for Fats - Monounsaturated

#12 Pork Liver

Total Nutrient Score: 20.57
Overall Rank: 25 of 8990
Meat and Seafood Rank: 12 of 20
Serving Size: 3 oz (85 g)
Cooking preparation: cooked, braised
Calories: 140 | Carbs: 3.2 g

661% FDI for Vitamin B12
510% FDI for Vitamin A
190% FDI for Iron
144% FDI for Riboflavin (Vitamin B2)
104% FDI for Selenium
81% FDI for Pantothenic Acid (Vitamin B5)
60% FDI for Copper
52% FDI for Zinc
45% FDI for Niacin (Vitamin B3)
37% FDI for Vitamin B6
35% FDI for Folate
29% FDI for Phosphorus
22% FDI for Vitamin C
22% FDI for Protein
18% FDI for Thiamine (Vitamin B1)
12% FDI for Omega-3 (DHA, 22:6)
11% FDI for Manganese
9% FDI for Fats - Polyunsaturated
4% FDI for Fats - Saturated
3% FDI for Magnesium
3% FDI for Potassium
1% FDI for Carbohydrate
1% FDI for Fats - Monounsaturated

#13 Pork Kidney

Total Nutrient Score: 19.97
Overall Rank: 27 of 8990
Meat and Seafood Rank: 13 of 20
Serving Size: 1 cup (140 g)
Cooking preparation: cooked, braised
Calories: 211 | Carbs: 0 g

793% FDI for Selenium *UL used for ranking analysis
455% FDI for Vitamin B12
171% FDI for Riboflavin (Vitamin B2)
106% FDI for Copper
93% FDI for Iron
80% FDI for Pantothenic Acid (Vitamin B5)
53% FDI for Zinc
51% FDI for Niacin (Vitamin B3)
50% FDI for Vitamin B6
48% FDI for Phosphorus
46% FDI for Thiamine (Vitamin B1)
36% FDI for Protein
16% FDI for Vitamin C
14% FDI for Folate
12% FDI for Vitamin A
9% FDI for Manganese
8% FDI for Fats - Saturated
6% FDI for Magnesium
5% FDI for Fats - Polyunsaturated
5% FDI for Fats - Monounsaturated
4% FDI for Potassium
2% FDI for Calcium

#14 Sardines

Total Nutrient Score: 19.80
Overall Rank: 28 of 8990
Meat and Seafood Rank: 14 of 20
Serving Size: 1 cup, drained (149 g)
Cooking preparation: canned in oil, drained solids with bone
Calories: 310 | Carbs: 0 g

555% FDI for Vitamin B12
345% FDI for Omega-3 (DHA, 22:6)
320% FDI for Omega-3 (EPA, 20:5)
143% FDI for Selenium
104% FDI for Phosphorus
77% FDI for Fats - Polyunsaturated
57% FDI for Calcium
54% FDI for Iron
49% FDI for Niacin (Vitamin B3)
37% FDI for Protein
31% FDI for Copper
26% FDI for Riboflavin (Vitamin B2)
20% FDI for Choline
20% FDI for Vitamin E
19% FDI for Vitamin B6
19% FDI for Pantothenic Acid (Vitamin B5)
18% FDI for Zinc
14% FDI for Fats - Monounsaturated
14% FDI for Magnesium
13% FDI for Potassium
10% FDI for Thiamine (Vitamin B1)
8% FDI for Fats - Saturated
7% FDI for Manganese
6% FDI for Vitamin D3
5% FDI for Vitamin A
5% FDI for Vitamin K1
4% FDI for Folate

#15 Octopus

Total Nutrient Score: 19.61
Overall Rank: 31 of 8990
Meat and Seafood Rank: 15 of 20
Serving Size: 3 oz (85 g)
Cooking preparation: cooked, moist heat
Calories: 139 | Carbs: 3.74 g

1275% FDI for Vitamin B12
139% FDI for Selenium
101% FDI for Iron
70% FDI for Copper
63% FDI for Omega-3 (DHA, 22:6)
59% FDI for Omega-3 (EPA, 20:5)
42% FDI for Vitamin B6
34% FDI for Phosphorus
26% FDI for Zinc
25% FDI for Protein
20% FDI for Niacin (Vitamin B3)
15% FDI for Pantothenic Acid (Vitamin B5)
13% FDI for Choline
12% FDI for Magnesium
11% FDI for Potassium
9% FDI for Calcium
9% FDI for Vitamin A
8% FDI for Vitamin C
7% FDI for Vitamin E
5% FDI for Folate
5% FDI for Riboflavin (Vitamin B2)
4% FDI for Fats – Polyunsaturated
4% FDI for Thiamine (Vitamin B1)
2% FDI for Manganese
2% FDI for Carbohydrate
1% FDI for Fats – Saturated

#16 Turkey Liver

Total Nutrient Score: 19.01
Overall Rank: 33 of 8990
Meat and Seafood Rank: 16 of 20
Serving Size: 1 liver cooked (53 g)
Cooking preparation: cooked, simmered
Calories: 100 | Carbs: 0 g

633% FDI for Vitamin A
622% FDI for Vitamin B12
110% FDI for Riboflavin (Vitamin B2)
99% FDI for Selenium
92% FDI for Folate
62% FDI for Copper
46% FDI for Pantothenic Acid (Vitamin B5)
37% FDI for Niacin (Vitamin B3)
36% FDI for Vitamin B6
24% FDI for Phosphorus
22% FDI for Zinc
21% FDI for Choline
14% FDI for Protein
13% FDI for Vitamin C
13% FDI for Omega-3 (DHA, 22:6)
12% FDI for Iron
11% FDI for Fats – Polyunsaturated
11% FDI for Thiamine (Vitamin B1)
8% FDI for Manganese
5% FDI for Fats – Saturated
4% FDI for Omega-3 (EPA, 20:5)
3% FDI for Magnesium
2% FDI for Potassium
1% FDI for Fats – Monounsaturated
1% FDI for Calcium

#17 Turkey Giblets

Total Nutrient Score: 18.69
Overall Rank: 35 of 8990
Meat and Seafood Rank: 17 of 20
Serving Size: 1 giblets (95 g)
Cooking preparation: cooked, simmered
Calories: 164 | Carbs: 0 g

629% FDI for Vitamin B12
488% FDI for Vitamin A
123% FDI for Selenium
113% FDI for Riboflavin (Vitamin B2)
73% FDI for Copper
72% FDI for Folate
51% FDI for Niacin (Vitamin B3)
44% FDI for Pantothenic Acid (Vitamin B5)
40% FDI for Iron
40% FDI for Vitamin B6
37% FDI for Zinc
34% FDI for Phosphorus
27% FDI for Choline
25% FDI for Protein
15% FDI for Fats - Polyunsaturated
14% FDI for Thiamine (Vitamin B1)
12% FDI for Omega-3 (DHA, 22:6)
8% FDI for Manganese
6% FDI for Fats - Saturated
6% FDI for Magnesium
5% FDI for Omega-3 (EPA, 20:5)
4% FDI for Potassium
2% FDI for Fats - Monounsaturated
2% FDI for Calcium

#18 Mussels

Total Nutrient Score: 18.61
Overall Rank: 36 of 8990
Meat and Seafood Rank: 18 of 20
Serving Size: 3 oz (85 g)
Cooking preparation: cooked, moist heat
Calories: 146 | Carbs: 6.28 g

850% FDI for Vitamin B12
251% FDI for Manganese
195% FDI for Omega-3 (DHA, 22:6)
139% FDI for Selenium
107% FDI for Omega-3 (EPA, 20:5)
71% FDI for Iron
35% FDI for Phosphorus
27% FDI for Riboflavin (Vitamin B2)
21% FDI for Thiamine (Vitamin B1)
21% FDI for Zinc
20% FDI for Protein
16% FDI for Folate
16% FDI for Pantothenic Acid (Vitamin B5)
16% FDI for Niacin (Vitamin B3)
14% FDI for Copper
13% FDI for Vitamin C
10% FDI for Fats - Polyunsaturated
9% FDI for Vitamin A
7% FDI for Magnesium
7% FDI for Vitamin B6
5% FDI for Potassium
3% FDI for Calcium
3% FDI for Carbohydrate
3% FDI for Fats - Saturated
2% FDI for Fats - Monounsaturated

#19 Beef Kidney

Total Nutrient Score: 17.44
Overall Rank: 40 of 8990
Meat and Seafood Rank: 19 of 20
Serving Size: 3 oz (85 g)
Cooking preparation: cooked, simmered
Calories: 134 | Carbs: 0 g

882% FDI for Vitamin B12
260% FDI for Selenium
194% FDI for Riboflavin (Vitamin B2)
79% FDI for Choline
62% FDI for Iron
53% FDI for Copper
37% FDI for Phosphorus
27% FDI for Pantothenic Acid (Vitamin B5)
26% FDI for Vitamin B6
23% FDI for Protein
22% FDI for Zinc
21% FDI for Niacin (Vitamin B3)
18% FDI for Folate
11% FDI for Thiamine (Vitamin B1)
10% FDI for Fats - Polyunsaturated
7% FDI for Manganese
5% FDI for Fats - Saturated
2% FDI for Potassium
2% FDI for Magnesium
2% FDI for Fats - Monounsaturated
2% FDI for Calcium

#20 Lamb Brain

Total Nutrient Score: 17.10
Overall Rank: 43 of 8990
Meat and Seafood Rank: 20 of 20
Serving Size: 3 oz (85 g)
Cooking preparation: cooked, pan-fried
Calories: 232 | Carbs: 0 g

853% FDI for Vitamin B12
495% FDI for Omega-3 (DHA, 22:6)
60% FDI for Phosphorus
45% FDI for Copper
27% FDI for Pantothenic Acid (Vitamin B5)
24% FDI for Niacin (Vitamin B3)
24% FDI for Riboflavin (Vitamin B2)
22% FDI for Vitamin C
22% FDI for Iron
19% FDI for Fats - Polyunsaturated
19% FDI for Selenium
18% FDI for Fats - Saturated
15% FDI for Zinc
15% FDI for Vitamin B6
14% FDI for Protein
12% FDI for Thiamine (Vitamin B1)
9% FDI for Fats - Monounsaturated
6% FDI for Potassium
5% FDI for Magnesium
2% FDI for Manganese
2% FDI for Calcium
2% FDI for Folate

VEGETABLES

Nutrients per One Serving

#1 Spinach (cooked or canned)

Total Nutrient Score: 29.80
Overall Rank: 6 of 8990
Vegetables Rank: 1 of 20
Serving Size: 1 cup (180 g)
Cooking preparation: cooked, boiled, drained, without salt
Calories: 41 | Carbs: 6.75 g

1111% FDI for Vitamin K1
629% FDI for Vitamin A
485% FDI for Lutein+Zeaxanthin
226% FDI for Beta-Carotene
80% FDI for Iron
73% FDI for Manganese
66% FDI for Folate
37% FDI for Magnesium
35% FDI for Copper
34% FDI for Vitamin B6
33% FDI for Riboflavin (Vitamin B2)
25% FDI for Vitamin E
25% FDI for Calcium
20% FDI for Vitamin C
18% FDI for Potassium
14% FDI for Phosphorus
14% FDI for Thiamine (Vitamin B1)
12% FDI for Zinc
11% FDI for Fiber
6% FDI for Choline
6% FDI for Niacin (Vitamin B3)
5% FDI for Protein
5% FDI for Pantothenic Acid (Vitamin B5)
5% FDI for Selenium
3% FDI for Carbohydrate
2% FDI for Fats - Polyunsaturated

#2 Kale

Total Nutrient Score: 29.05
Overall Rank: 7 of 8990
Vegetables Rank: 2 of 20
Serving Size: 1 cup, chopped (130 g)
Cooking preparation: cooked, boiled, drained, without salt
Calories: 36 | Carbs: 7.32 g

1328% FDI for Vitamin K1
590% FDI for Vitamin A
565% FDI for Lutein+Zeaxanthin
213% FDI for Beta-Carotene
59% FDI for Vitamin C
24% FDI for Manganese
23% FDI for Copper
15% FDI for Iron
14% FDI for Vitamin B6
9% FDI for Calcium
7% FDI for Vitamin E
7% FDI for Riboflavin (Vitamin B2)
7% FDI for Fiber
6% FDI for Potassium
6% FDI for Thiamine (Vitamin B1)
5% FDI for Magnesium
5% FDI for Phosphorus
4% FDI for Folate
4% FDI for Niacin (Vitamin B3)
3% FDI for Carbohydrate
3% FDI for Zinc
3% FDI for Fats - Polyunsaturated
2% FDI for Protein
2% FDI for Selenium
1% FDI for Pantothenic Acid (Vitamin B5)

#3 Sweet Potato

Total Nutrient Score: 27.63
Overall Rank: 11 of 8990
Vegetables Rank: 3 of 20
Serving Size: 1 cup, mashed (328 g)
Cooking preparation: cooked, boiled, without skin
Calories: 249 | Carbs: 58.12 g

1721% FDI for Vitamin A
620% FDI for Beta-Carotene
47% FDI for Vitamin C
42% FDI for Vitamin B6
38% FDI for Pantothenic Acid (Vitamin B5)
38% FDI for Manganese
34% FDI for Copper
30% FDI for Iron
26% FDI for Carbohydrate
22% FDI for Fiber
21% FDI for Vitamin E
16% FDI for Potassium
15% FDI for Thiamine (Vitamin B1)
15% FDI for Phosphorus
14% FDI for Magnesium
12% FDI for Riboflavin (Vitamin B2)
11% FDI for Niacin (Vitamin B3)
9% FDI for Calcium
9% FDI for Vitamin K1
6% FDI for Choline
6% FDI for Zinc
5% FDI for Folate
4% FDI for Protein
2% FDI for Fats - Polyunsaturated
1% FDI for Selenium

#4 Pumpkin (canned)

Total Nutrient Score: 27.03
Overall Rank: 12 of 8990
Vegetables Rank: 4 of 20
Serving Size: 1 cup (245 g)
Cooking preparation: canned, without salt
Calories: 83 | Carbs: 19.82 g

1271% FDI for Vitamin A
783% FDI for Alpha-Carotene
340% FDI for Beta-Carotene
49% FDI for Vitamin K1
43% FDI for Iron
29% FDI for Copper
20% FDI for Pantothenic Acid (Vitamin B5)
19% FDI for Fiber
17% FDI for Vitamin E
16% FDI for Manganese
13% FDI for Magnesium
12% FDI for Phosphorus
11% FDI for Vitamin C
11% FDI for Potassium
11% FDI for Vitamin B6
10% FDI for Riboflavin (Vitamin B2)
9% FDI for Carbohydrate
7% FDI for Folate
6% FDI for Calcium
6% FDI for Niacin (Vitamin B3)
5% FDI for Thiamine (Vitamin B1)
4% FDI for Choline
4% FDI for Zinc
3% FDI for Protein
2% FDI for Selenium
1% FDI for Fats - Saturated

#5 Butternut Squash

Total Nutrient Score: 25.69
Overall Rank: 14 of 8990
Vegetables Rank: 5 of 20
Serving Size: 1 cup, cubes (205 g)
Cooking preparation: cooked, baked, without salt
Calories: 82 | Carbs: 21.5 g

1217% FDI for Beta-Cryptoxanthin
762% FDI for Vitamin A
187% FDI for Beta-Carotene
154% FDI for Alpha-Carotene
34% FDI for Vitamin C
20% FDI for Vitamin B6
18% FDI for Vitamin E
17% FDI for Fiber
15% FDI for Iron
15% FDI for Manganese
15% FDI for Copper
15% FDI for Pantothenic Acid (Vitamin B5)
14% FDI for Magnesium
12% FDI for Niacin (Vitamin B3)
12% FDI for Potassium
12% FDI for Thiamine (Vitamin B1)
10% FDI for Folate
10% FDI for Carbohydrate
8% FDI for Calcium
8% FDI for Phosphorus
3% FDI for Riboflavin (Vitamin B2)
3% FDI for Vitamin K1
2% FDI for Zinc
2% FDI for Protein
2% FDI for Selenium

#6 Seaweed, Spirulina (dried)

Total Nutrient Score: 24.17
Overall Rank: 17 of 8990
Vegetables Rank: 6 of 20
Serving Size: 1 cup (112 g)
Cooking preparation: dried
Calories: 325 | Carbs: 26.77 g

759% FDI for Copper
399% FDI for Iron
316% FDI for Riboflavin (Vitamin B2)
222% FDI for Thiamine (Vitamin B1)
93% FDI for Manganese
90% FDI for Niacin (Vitamin B3)
78% FDI for Pantothenic Acid (Vitamin B5)
64% FDI for Protein
52% FDI for Magnesium
37% FDI for Vitamin E
36% FDI for Vitamin K1
32% FDI for Potassium
31% FDI for Vitamin B6
26% FDI for Folate
23% FDI for Fats – Polyunsaturated
21% FDI for Vitamin A
20% FDI for Zinc
19% FDI for Phosphorus
15% FDI for Selenium
13% FDI for Choline
13% FDI for Calcium
13% FDI for Vitamin C
12% FDI for Carbohydrate
11% FDI for Fats – Saturated
11% FDI for Fiber
8% FDI for Beta-Carotene
2% FDI for Fats – Monounsaturated

#7 Mustard Greens

Total Nutrient Score: 23.58
Overall Rank: 18 of 8990
Vegetables Rank: 7 of 20
Serving Size: 1 cup, chopped (140 g)
Cooking preparation: cooked, boiled, drained, without salt
Calories: 36 | Carbs: 6.31 g

1037% FDI for Vitamin K1
577% FDI for Vitamin A
347% FDI for Lutein+Zeaxanthin
207% FDI for Beta-Carotene
39% FDI for Vitamin C
23% FDI for Copper
17% FDI for Vitamin E
17% FDI for Calcium
15% FDI for Iron
11% FDI for Vitamin B6
9% FDI for Beta-Cryptoxanthin
8% FDI for Phosphorus
7% FDI for Fiber
7% FDI for Riboflavin (Vitamin B2)
5% FDI for Potassium
5% FDI for Thiamine (Vitamin B1)
4% FDI for Magnesium
4% FDI for Niacin (Vitamin B3)
4% FDI for Protein
3% FDI for Pantothenic Acid (Vitamin B5)
3% FDI for Folate
3% FDI for Zinc
3% FDI for Carbohydrate
1% FDI for Selenium

#8 Lambsquarters

Total Nutrient Score: 22.29
Overall Rank: 19 of 8990
Vegetables Rank: 8 of 20
Serving Size: 1 cup, chopped (180 g)
Cooking preparation: cooked, boiled, drained, without salt
Calories: 58 | Carbs: 9 g

1112% FDI for Vitamin K1
469% FDI for Vitamin A
169% FDI for Beta-Carotene
80% FDI for Lutein+Zeaxanthin
74% FDI for Vitamin C
46% FDI for Calcium
41% FDI for Manganese
39% FDI for Copper
36% FDI for Riboflavin (Vitamin B2)
24% FDI for Vitamin B6
22% FDI for Vitamin E
16% FDI for Iron
15% FDI for Thiamine (Vitamin B1)
12% FDI for Phosphorus
11% FDI for Potassium
10% FDI for Niacin (Vitamin B3)
10% FDI for Fiber
10% FDI for Magnesium
6% FDI for Folate
6% FDI for Protein
6% FDI for Fats – Polyunsaturated
5% FDI for Zinc
4% FDI for Carbohydrate
3% FDI for Selenium
2% FDI for Pantothenic Acid (Vitamin B5)

#9 Collard Greens

Total Nutrient Score: 22.12
Overall Rank: 21 of 8990
Vegetables Rank: 9 of 20
Serving Size: 1 cup, chopped (190 g)
Cooking preparation: cooked, boiled, drained, without salt
Calories: 63 | Carbs: 10.74 g

966% FDI for Vitamin K1
481% FDI for Vitamin A
280% FDI for Lutein+Zeaxanthin
172% FDI for Beta-Carotene
42% FDI for Manganese
38% FDI for Vitamin C
27% FDI for Iron
27% FDI for Calcium
20% FDI for Fiber
19% FDI for Vitamin B6
15% FDI for Riboflavin (Vitamin B2)
13% FDI for Choline
11% FDI for Vitamin E
11% FDI for Copper
10% FDI for Magnesium
9% FDI for Beta-Cryptoxanthin
9% FDI for Phosphorus
9% FDI for Alpha-Carotene
8% FDI for Pantothenic Acid (Vitamin B5)
8% FDI for Folate
7% FDI for Niacin (Vitamin B3)
6% FDI for Thiamine (Vitamin B1)
5% FDI for Protein
5% FDI for Carbohydrate
5% FDI for Potassium
4% FDI for Zinc
3% FDI for Fats - Polyunsaturated
2% FDI for Selenium

#10 Swiss Chard

Total Nutrient Score: 19.79
Overall Rank: 29 of 8990
Vegetables Rank: 10 of 20
Serving Size: 1 cup, chopped (175 g)
Cooking preparation: cooked, boiled, drained, without salt
Calories: 35 | Carbs: 7.23 g

716% FDI for Vitamin K1
459% FDI for Lutein+Zeaxanthin
357% FDI for Vitamin A
128% FDI for Beta-Carotene
49% FDI for Iron
36% FDI for Magnesium
35% FDI for Vitamin C
32% FDI for Copper
25% FDI for Manganese
22% FDI for Vitamin E
20% FDI for Potassium
12% FDI for Riboflavin (Vitamin B2)
11% FDI for Vitamin B6
10% FDI for Calcium
10% FDI for Fiber
9% FDI for Choline
8% FDI for Phosphorus
6% FDI for Pantothenic Acid (Vitamin B5)
5% FDI for Zinc
5% FDI for Alpha-Carotene
5% FDI for Thiamine (Vitamin B1)
4% FDI for Folate
4% FDI for Niacin (Vitamin B3)
3% FDI for Protein
3% FDI for Carbohydrate
3% FDI for Selenium

#11 Beet Greens

Total Nutrient Score: 17.82
Overall Rank: 37 of 8990
Vegetables Rank: 11 of 20
Serving Size: 1 cup (1" pieces) (144 g)
Cooking preparation: cooked, boiled, drained, without salt
Calories: 39 | Carbs: 7.86 g

871% FDI for Vitamin K1
367% FDI for Vitamin A
132% FDI for Beta-Carotene
62% FDI for Lutein+Zeaxanthin
40% FDI for Copper
40% FDI for Vitamin C
34% FDI for Iron
32% FDI for Manganese
32% FDI for Riboflavin (Vitamin B2)
28% FDI for Potassium
23% FDI for Magnesium
17% FDI for Vitamin E
16% FDI for Calcium
15% FDI for Vitamin B6
14% FDI for Thiamine (Vitamin B1)
11% FDI for Fiber
9% FDI for Pantothenic Acid (Vitamin B5)
8% FDI for Phosphorus
7% FDI for Zinc
5% FDI for Folate
4% FDI for Niacin (Vitamin B3)
4% FDI for Protein
3% FDI for Carbohydrate
2% FDI for Selenium
1% FDI for Fats – Polyunsaturated

#12 Parsley

Total Nutrient Score: 17.81
Overall Rank: 38 of 8990
Vegetables Rank: 12 of 20
Serving Size: 1 cup chopped (60 g)
Cooking preparation: fresh
Calories: 22 | Carbs: 3.8 g

1230% FDI for Vitamin K1
168% FDI for Vitamin A
89% FDI for Vitamin C
79% FDI for Lutein+Zeaxanthin
61% FDI for Beta-Carotene
47% FDI for Iron
23% FDI for Folate
10% FDI for Copper
8% FDI for Calcium
7% FDI for Magnesium
7% FDI for Potassium
6% FDI for Zinc
5% FDI for Fiber
5% FDI for Phosphorus
5% FDI for Niacin (Vitamin B3)
5% FDI for Pantothenic Acid (Vitamin B5)
5% FDI for Riboflavin (Vitamin B2)
4% FDI for Thiamine (Vitamin B1)
4% FDI for Manganese
4% FDI for Vitamin B6
3% FDI for Vitamin E
2% FDI for Protein
2% FDI for Carbohydrate
1% FDI for Choline

#13 Turnip Greens

Total Nutrient Score: 17.37
Overall Rank: 41 of 8990
Vegetables Rank: 13 of 20
Serving Size: 1 cup, chopped (144 g)
Cooking preparation: cooked, boiled, drained, without salt
Calories: 29 | Carbs: 6.28 g

662% FDI for Vitamin K1
366% FDI for Vitamin A
289% FDI for Lutein+Zeaxanthin
132% FDI for Beta-Carotene
44% FDI for Vitamin C
43% FDI for Folate
40% FDI for Copper
21% FDI for Manganese
20% FDI for Vitamin B6
20% FDI for Calcium
18% FDI for Vitamin E
14% FDI for Iron
13% FDI for Fiber
8% FDI for Riboflavin (Vitamin B2)
8% FDI for Pantothenic Acid (Vitamin B5)
8% FDI for Magnesium
6% FDI for Potassium
6% FDI for Phosphorus
5% FDI for Thiamine (Vitamin B1)
4% FDI for Niacin (Vitamin B3)
3% FDI for Carbohydrate
2% FDI for Selenium
2% FDI for Zinc
2% FDI for Protein
2% FDI for Fats - Polyunsaturated

#14 Dandelion Greens

Total Nutrient Score: 14.97
Overall Rank: 48 of 8990
Vegetables Rank: 14 of 20
Serving Size: 1 cup, chopped (105 g)
Cooking preparation: cooked, boiled, drained, without salt
Calories: 35 | Carbs: 6.72 g

724% FDI for Vitamin K1
239% FDI for Vitamin A
229% FDI for Lutein+Zeaxanthin
83% FDI for Beta-Carotene
24% FDI for Iron
21% FDI for Vitamin C
17% FDI for Vitamin E
17% FDI for Alpha-Carotene
16% FDI for Beta-Cryptoxanthin
15% FDI for Calcium
14% FDI for Riboflavin (Vitamin B2)
13% FDI for Copper
13% FDI for Vitamin B6
11% FDI for Thiamine (Vitamin B1)
11% FDI for Manganese
8% FDI for Fiber
6% FDI for Phosphorus
6% FDI for Magnesium
5% FDI for Potassium
5% FDI for Choline
4% FDI for Folate
3% FDI for Niacin (Vitamin B3)
3% FDI for Carbohydrate
3% FDI for Fats - Polyunsaturated
3% FDI for Zinc
2% FDI for Protein
1% FDI for Pantothenic Acid (Vitamin B5)

#15 Garden Cress

Total Nutrient Score: 14.10
Overall Rank: 58 of 8990
Vegetables Rank: 15 of 20
Serving Size: 1 cup (135 g)
Cooking preparation: cooked, boiled, drained, without salt
Calories: 31 | Carbs: 5.13 g

647% FDI for Vitamin K1
270% FDI for Lutein+Zeaxanthin
209% FDI for Vitamin A
75% FDI for Beta-Carotene
34% FDI for Vitamin C
22% FDI for Manganese
17% FDI for Copper
17% FDI for Riboflavin (Vitamin B2)
16% FDI for Vitamin B6
14% FDI for Iron
13% FDI for Folate
10% FDI for Potassium
9% FDI for Phosphorus
8% FDI for Magnesium
8% FDI for Calcium
7% FDI for Niacin (Vitamin B3)
7% FDI for Thiamine (Vitamin B1)
5% FDI for Vitamin E
4% FDI for Pantothenic Acid (Vitamin B5)
3% FDI for Choline
3% FDI for Fats - Polyunsaturated
3% FDI for Protein
2% FDI for Fiber
2% FDI for Carbohydrate
2% FDI for Selenium
2% FDI for Zinc

#16 Carrots

Total Nutrient Score: 13.77
Overall Rank: 65 of 8990
Vegetables Rank: 16 of 20
Serving Size: 1 cup chopped (128 g)
Cooking preparation: raw
Calories: 52 | Carbs: 12.26 g

713% FDI for Vitamin A
297% FDI for Alpha-Carotene
212% FDI for Beta-Carotene
21% FDI for Vitamin K1
14% FDI for Vitamin B6
9% FDI for Fiber
9% FDI for Potassium
8% FDI for Vitamin C
8% FDI for Manganese
8% FDI for Niacin (Vitamin B3)
8% FDI for Lutein+Zeaxanthin
7% FDI for Thiamine (Vitamin B1)
7% FDI for Pantothenic Acid (Vitamin B5)
6% FDI for Copper
6% FDI for Phosphorus
6% FDI for Folate
6% FDI for Riboflavin (Vitamin B2)
6% FDI for Vitamin E
5% FDI for Carbohydrate
5% FDI for Iron
4% FDI for Calcium
4% FDI for Magnesium
3% FDI for Zinc
2% FDI for Choline
2% FDI for Fats - Polyunsaturated
1% FDI for Protein

#17 Pokeberry Shoots

Total Nutrient Score: 12.96
Overall Rank: 69 of 8990
Vegetables Rank: 17 of 20
Serving Size: 1 cup (165 g)
Cooking preparation: cooked, boiled, drained, without salt
Calories: 33 | Carbs: 5.12 g

479% FDI for Vitamin A
223% FDI for Vitamin K1
172% FDI for Beta-Carotene
150% FDI for Vitamin C
69% FDI for Lutein+Zeaxanthin
32% FDI for Riboflavin (Vitamin B2)
25% FDI for Iron
24% FDI for Manganese
23% FDI for Copper
14% FDI for Vitamin B6
11% FDI for Niacin (Vitamin B3)
10% FDI for Thiamine (Vitamin B1)
9% FDI for Vitamin E
9% FDI for Calcium
8% FDI for Phosphorus
7% FDI for Fiber
6% FDI for Potassium
5% FDI for Magnesium
4% FDI for Protein
4% FDI for Folate
3% FDI for Fats - Polyunsaturated
3% FDI for Zinc
3% FDI for Selenium
2% FDI for Carbohydrate
1% FDI for Pantothenic Acid (Vitamin B5)

#18 Pumpkin

Total Nutrient Score: 12.61
Overall Rank: 72 of 8990
Vegetables Rank: 18 of 20
Serving Size: 1 cup, mashed (245 g)
Cooking preparation: cooked, boiled, drained, without salt
Calories: 49 | Carbs: 12 g

470% FDI for Vitamin A
443% FDI for Alpha-Carotene
103% FDI for Beta-Carotene
59% FDI for Lutein+Zeaxanthin
25% FDI for Copper
18% FDI for Iron
15% FDI for Riboflavin (Vitamin B2)
13% FDI for Vitamin E
13% FDI for Vitamin C
12% FDI for Potassium
11% FDI for Phosphorus
10% FDI for Pantothenic Acid (Vitamin B5)
9% FDI for Manganese
8% FDI for Vitamin B6
7% FDI for Fiber
6% FDI for Thiamine (Vitamin B1)
6% FDI for Niacin (Vitamin B3)
6% FDI for Folate
5% FDI for Carbohydrate
5% FDI for Magnesium
5% FDI for Zinc
4% FDI for Calcium
3% FDI for Choline
3% FDI for Vitamin K1
2% FDI for Protein

#19 Hubbard Squash

Total Nutrient Score: 11.37
Overall Rank: 90 of 8990
Vegetables Rank: 19 of 20
Serving Size: 1 cup, mashed (236 g)
Cooking preparation: cooked, boiled, mashed, without salt
Calories: 71 | Carbs: 15.25 g

503% FDI for Beta-Cryptoxanthin
315% FDI for Vitamin A
77% FDI for Beta-Carotene
64% FDI for Alpha-Carotene
19% FDI for Vitamin B6
18% FDI for Fiber
17% FDI for Vitamin C
14% FDI for Pantothenic Acid (Vitamin B5)
13% FDI for Manganese
12% FDI for Copper
11% FDI for Potassium
8% FDI for Iron
8% FDI for Thiamine (Vitamin B1)
7% FDI for Magnesium
7% FDI for Carbohydrate
6% FDI for Folate
5% FDI for Riboflavin (Vitamin B2)
5% FDI for Niacin (Vitamin B3)
5% FDI for Phosphorus
4% FDI for Choline
4% FDI for Fats – Polyunsaturated
3% FDI for Protein
3% FDI for Vitamin K1
2% FDI for Calcium
2% FDI for Zinc
2% FDI for Vitamin E
1% FDI for Selenium

#20 Radishes (dried)

Total Nutrient Score: 10.44
Overall Rank: 112 of 8990
Vegetables Rank: 20 of 20
Serving Size: 1 cup (116 g)
Cooking preparation: dried
Calories: 314 | Carbs: 73.51 g

210% FDI for Copper
98% FDI for Iron
86% FDI for Potassium
86% FDI for Folate
73% FDI for Calcium
73% FDI for Fiber
61% FDI for Riboflavin (Vitamin B2)
55% FDI for Vitamin B6
47% FDI for Magnesium
43% FDI for Pantothenic Acid (Vitamin B5)
34% FDI for Phosphorus
33% FDI for Carbohydrate
27% FDI for Manganese
26% FDI for Thiamine (Vitamin B1)
25% FDI for Niacin (Vitamin B3)
23% FDI for Choline
22% FDI for Zinc
9% FDI for Protein
7% FDI for Vitamin K1
4% FDI for Fats – Polyunsaturated
1% FDI for Selenium

FRUITS

Nutrients per One Serving

#1 Acerola Cherry

Total Nutrient Score: 19.03
Overall Rank: 32 of 8990
Fruit Rank: 1 of 20
Serving Size: 1 cup (98 g)
Calories: 31 | Carbs: 7.54 g

1827% FDI for Vitamin C
25% FDI for Vitamin A
9% FDI for Copper
6% FDI for Pantothenic Acid (Vitamin B5)
5% FDI for Riboflavin (Vitamin B2)
4% FDI for Magnesium
4% FDI for Folate
3% FDI for Carbohydrate
3% FDI for Potassium
3% FDI for Fiber
3% FDI for Iron
2% FDI for Niacin (Vitamin B3)
2% FDI for Thiamine (Vitamin B1)
2% FDI for Phosphorus
1% FDI for Calcium
1% FDI for Fats - Polyunsaturated
1% FDI for Selenium

#2 Rose Hips

Total Nutrient Score: 15.23
Overall Rank: 46 of 8990
Fruit Rank: 2 of 20
Serving Size: 1 cup (127 g)
Calories: 206 | Carbs: 48.54 g

601% FDI for Vitamin C
184% FDI for Vitamin A
117% FDI for Beta-Cryptoxanthin
86% FDI for Lycopene
81% FDI for Fiber
61% FDI for Lutein+Zeaxanthin
60% FDI for Beta-Carotene
56% FDI for Manganese
49% FDI for Vitamin E
41% FDI for Vitamin K1
22% FDI for Carbohydrate
22% FDI for Calcium
21% FDI for Magnesium
20% FDI for Pantothenic Acid (Vitamin B5)
17% FDI for Iron
16% FDI for Riboflavin (Vitamin B2)
16% FDI for Copper
12% FDI for Potassium
11% FDI for Phosphorus
10% FDI for Niacin (Vitamin B3)
7% FDI for Vitamin B6
3% FDI for Zinc
3% FDI for Choline
3% FDI for Alpha-Carotene
2% FDI for Protein
2% FDI for Thiamine (Vitamin B1)
1% FDI for Folate

#3 Peaches (dried)

Total Nutrient Score: 7.98
Overall Rank: 187 of 8990
Fruit Rank: 3 of 20
Serving Size: 1 cup, halves (160 g)
Calories: 382 | Carbs: 98.13 g

135% FDI for Beta-Cryptoxanthin
115% FDI for Vitamin A
81% FDI for Iron
65% FDI for Copper
44% FDI for Niacin (Vitamin B3)
44% FDI for Carbohydrate
34% FDI for Fiber
34% FDI for Beta-Carotene
34% FDI for Potassium
31% FDI for Vitamin K1
27% FDI for Phosphorus
26% FDI for Riboflavin (Vitamin B2)
21% FDI for Lutein+Zeaxanthin
21% FDI for Manganese
18% FDI for Pantothenic Acid (Vitamin B5)
16% FDI for Magnesium
9% FDI for Vitamin C
8% FDI for Zinc
8% FDI for Vitamin B6
6% FDI for Fats – Polyunsaturated
6% FDI for Protein
5% FDI for Calcium
4% FDI for Choline
2% FDI for Vitamin E
1% FDI for Selenium
1% FDI for Fats – Monounsaturated

#4 Guavas

Total Nutrient Score: 7.87
Overall Rank: 190 of 8990
Fruit Rank: 4 of 20
Serving Size: 1 cup (165 g)
Calories: 112 | Carbs: 23.63 g

419% FDI for Vitamin C
86% FDI for Lycopene
42% FDI for Copper
34% FDI for Vitamin A
23% FDI for Fiber
20% FDI for Folate
15% FDI for Pantothenic Acid (Vitamin B5)
15% FDI for Potassium
14% FDI for Vitamin B6
12% FDI for Beta-Carotene
11% FDI for Niacin (Vitamin B3)
11% FDI for Manganese
11% FDI for Carbohydrate
9% FDI for Phosphorus
9% FDI for Thiamine (Vitamin B1)
9% FDI for Magnesium
8% FDI for Vitamin E
7% FDI for Fats – Polyunsaturated
5% FDI for Vitamin K1
5% FDI for Iron
5% FDI for Riboflavin (Vitamin B2)
4% FDI for Protein
3% FDI for Zinc
3% FDI for Calcium
2% FDI for Choline
2% FDI for Selenium
2% FDI for Fats – Saturated

#5 Persimmons

Total Nutrient Score: 7.53
Overall Rank: 203 of 8990
Fruit Rank: 5 of 20
Serving Size: 1 fruit (2-1/2" diameter) (168 g)
Calories: 118 | Carbs: 31.23 g

463% FDI for Beta-Cryptoxanthin
91% FDI for Vitamin A
33% FDI for Lutein+Zeaxanthin
26% FDI for Manganese
21% FDI for Copper
16% FDI for Fiber
14% FDI for Vitamin C
14% FDI for Carbohydrate
13% FDI for Vitamin B6
9% FDI for Beta-Carotene
8% FDI for Vitamin E
6% FDI for Potassium
6% FDI for Vitamin K1
4% FDI for Thiamine (Vitamin B1)
4% FDI for Phosphorus
4% FDI for Magnesium
3% FDI for Folate
3% FDI for Iron
3% FDI for Lycopene
3% FDI for Riboflavin (Vitamin B2)
2% FDI for Choline
2% FDI for Selenium
2% FDI for Protein
2% FDI for Zinc
1% FDI for Calcium
1% FDI for Niacin (Vitamin B3)

#6 Mammy-Apple

Total Nutrient Score: 7.38
Overall Rank: 221 of 8990
Fruit Rank: 6 of 20
Serving Size: 1 fruit without refuse (846 g)
Calories: 431 | Carbs: 105.75 g

132% FDI for Vitamin C
81% FDI for Copper
74% FDI for Iron
67% FDI for Fiber
65% FDI for Vitamin B6
65% FDI for Vitamin A
47% FDI for Carbohydrate
32% FDI for Magnesium
30% FDI for Folate
26% FDI for Riboflavin (Vitamin B2)
21% FDI for Niacin (Vitamin B3)
17% FDI for Pantothenic Acid (Vitamin B5)
14% FDI for Thiamine (Vitamin B1)
13% FDI for Phosphorus
9% FDI for Calcium
9% FDI for Selenium
8% FDI for Potassium
8% FDI for Zinc
7% FDI for Fats - Polyunsaturated
4% FDI for Fats - Monounsaturated
4% FDI for Fats - Saturated
4% FDI for Protein

#7 Avocados

Total Nutrient Score: 7.24
Overall Rank: 241 of 8990
Fruit Rank: 7 of 20
Serving Size: 1 cup, pureed (230 g)
Calories: 384 | Carbs: 19.87 g

67% FDI for Pantothenic Acid (Vitamin B5)
60% FDI for Vitamin K1
56% FDI for Fats - Monounsaturated
51% FDI for Folate
51% FDI for Vitamin B6
43% FDI for Copper
42% FDI for Fats - Polyunsaturated
41% FDI for Fiber
30% FDI for Vitamin E
27% FDI for Niacin (Vitamin B3)
25% FDI for Riboflavin (Vitamin B2)
25% FDI for Potassium
22% FDI for Vitamin C
18% FDI for Fats - Saturated
18% FDI for Phosphorus
18% FDI for Iron
16% FDI for Magnesium
15% FDI for Manganese
15% FDI for Lutein+Zeaxanthin
14% FDI for Thiamine (Vitamin B1)
14% FDI for Zinc
12% FDI for Beta-Cryptoxanthin
11% FDI for Vitamin A
9% FDI for Carbohydrate
6% FDI for Choline
5% FDI for Protein
4% FDI for Alpha-Carotene
3% FDI for Calcium
3% FDI for Beta-Carotene
2% FDI for Selenium

#8 Prunes

Total Nutrient Score: 5.99
Overall Rank: 382 of 8990
Fruit Rank: 8 of 20
Serving Size: 1 cup, pitted (174 g)
Calories: 418 | Carbs: 111.15 g

129% FDI for Vitamin K1
54% FDI for Copper
49% FDI for Carbohydrate
45% FDI for Vitamin A
33% FDI for Fiber
31% FDI for Beta-Cryptoxanthin
27% FDI for Vitamin B6
27% FDI for Potassium
25% FDI for Riboflavin (Vitamin B2)
23% FDI for Manganese
20% FDI for Niacin (Vitamin B3)
20% FDI for Iron
17% FDI for Phosphorus
17% FDI for Magnesium
15% FDI for Pantothenic Acid (Vitamin B5)
14% FDI for Beta-Carotene
8% FDI for Calcium
7% FDI for Thiamine (Vitamin B1)
7% FDI for Zinc
7% FDI for Alpha-Carotene
6% FDI for Lutein+Zeaxanthin
5% FDI for Vitamin E
4% FDI for Protein
3% FDI for Choline
2% FDI for Folate
1% FDI for Vitamin C
1% FDI for Fats - Polyunsaturated

#9 Apricots (dried)

Total Nutrient Score: 5.66
Overall Rank: 438 of 8990
Fruit Rank: 9 of 20
Serving Size: 1 cup, halves (130 g)
Calories: 313 | Carbs: 81.43 g

156% FDI for Vitamin A
56% FDI for Beta-Carotene
50% FDI for Copper
43% FDI for Iron
38% FDI for Vitamin E
36% FDI for Carbohydrate
32% FDI for Potassium
25% FDI for Fiber
21% FDI for Niacin (Vitamin B3)
14% FDI for Vitamin B6
13% FDI for Pantothenic Acid (Vitamin B5)
13% FDI for Manganese
13% FDI for Phosphorus
10% FDI for Magnesium
7% FDI for Riboflavin (Vitamin B2)
7% FDI for Calcium
5% FDI for Selenium
5% FDI for Vitamin K1
5% FDI for Zinc
4% FDI for Protein
3% FDI for Choline
3% FDI for Folate
2% FDI for Thiamine (Vitamin B1)
1% FDI for Vitamin C
1% FDI for Fats - Polyunsaturated

#10 Passion-Fruit

Total Nutrient Score: 5.49
Overall Rank: 470 of 8990
Fruit Rank: 10 of 20
Serving Size: 1 cup (236 g)
Calories: 229 | Carbs: 55.18 g

100% FDI for Vitamin A
79% FDI for Vitamin C
64% FDI for Fiber
47% FDI for Iron
35% FDI for Beta-Carotene
25% FDI for Carbohydrate
24% FDI for Riboflavin (Vitamin B2)
23% FDI for Phosphorus
23% FDI for Copper
22% FDI for Niacin (Vitamin B3)
18% FDI for Beta-Cryptoxanthin
18% FDI for Vitamin B6
17% FDI for Potassium
16% FDI for Magnesium
10% FDI for Fats - Polyunsaturated
8% FDI for Folate
5% FDI for Protein
3% FDI for Choline
3% FDI for Calcium
3% FDI for Selenium
2% FDI for Zinc
2% FDI for Vitamin K1

#11 Plums

Total Nutrient Score: 5.08
Overall Rank: 574 of 8990
Fruit Rank: 11 of 20
Serving Size: 1 cup (161 g)
Calories: 147 | Carbs: 35.34 g

186% FDI for Vitamin A
62% FDI for Beta-Carotene
48% FDI for Beta-Cryptoxanthin
35% FDI for Lutein+Zeaxanthin
26% FDI for Fiber
23% FDI for Vitamin K1
18% FDI for Vitamin C
16% FDI for Carbohydrate
15% FDI for Alpha-Carotene
12% FDI for Potassium
12% FDI for Vitamin B6
10% FDI for Pantothenic Acid (Vitamin B5)
7% FDI for Phosphorus
6% FDI for Copper
6% FDI for Vitamin E
5% FDI for Manganese
5% FDI for Riboflavin (Vitamin B2)
4% FDI for Niacin (Vitamin B3)
3% FDI for Iron
3% FDI for Magnesium
2% FDI for Calcium
2% FDI for Choline
1% FDI for Zinc
1% FDI for Protein

#12 Durian

Total Nutrient Score: 5.02
Overall Rank: 603 of 8990
Fruit Rank: 12 of 20
Serving Size: 1 cup, chopped or diced (243 g)
Cooking preparation: raw or frozen
Calories: 357 | Carbs: 65.83 g

76% FDI for Thiamine (Vitamin B1)
59% FDI for Vitamin B6
56% FDI for Copper
53% FDI for Vitamin C
37% FDI for Riboflavin (Vitamin B2)
34% FDI for Manganese
29% FDI for Carbohydrate
24% FDI for Fiber
23% FDI for Potassium
22% FDI for Folate
17% FDI for Magnesium
16% FDI for Niacin (Vitamin B3)
14% FDI for Phosphorus
13% FDI for Iron
11% FDI for Pantothenic Acid (Vitamin B5)
6% FDI for Zinc
4% FDI for Protein
4% FDI for Vitamin A
2% FDI for Calcium
1% FDI for Beta-Carotene
1% FDI for Alpha-Carotene

#13 Kiwi

Total Nutrient Score: 4.58
Overall Rank: 802 of 8990
Fruit Rank: 13 of 20
Serving Size: 1 cup, sliced (180 g)
Calories: 110 | Carbs: 26.39 g

185% FDI for Vitamin C
91% FDI for Vitamin K1
26% FDI for Copper
18% FDI for Vitamin E
14% FDI for Fiber
12% FDI for Potassium
12% FDI for Carbohydrate
11% FDI for Folate
9% FDI for Phosphorus
9% FDI for Vitamin B6
8% FDI for Manganese
7% FDI for Magnesium
7% FDI for Iron
7% FDI for Pantothenic Acid (Vitamin B5)
6% FDI for Calcium
5% FDI for Lutein+Zeaxanthin
5% FDI for Vitamin A
5% FDI for Fats - Polyunsaturated
4% FDI for Thiamine (Vitamin B1)
4% FDI for Niacin (Vitamin B3)
3% FDI for Riboflavin (Vitamin B2)
3% FDI for Choline
2% FDI for Zinc
2% FDI for Protein
2% FDI for Beta-Carotene

#14 Cantaloupe

Total Nutrient Score: 4.49
Overall Rank: 858 of 8990
Fruit Rank: 14 of 20
Serving Size: 1 cup, balls (177 g)
Calories: 60 | Carbs: 14.44 g

200% FDI for Vitamin A
72% FDI for Vitamin C
72% FDI for Beta-Carotene
10% FDI for Potassium
10% FDI for Vitamin B6
9% FDI for Folate
8% FDI for Niacin (Vitamin B3)
8% FDI for Copper
6% FDI for Carbohydrate
6% FDI for Thiamine (Vitamin B1)
6% FDI for Vitamin K1
5% FDI for Magnesium
5% FDI for Iron
4% FDI for Fiber
4% FDI for Phosphorus
4% FDI for Pantothenic Acid (Vitamin B5)
3% FDI for Manganese
3% FDI for Zinc
3% FDI for Riboflavin (Vitamin B2)
2% FDI for Choline
2% FDI for Alpha-Carotene
2% FDI for Calcium
1% FDI for Protein
1% FDI for Fats - Polyunsaturated
1% FDI for Selenium
1% FDI for Lutein+Zeaxanthin

#14 Currants (dried)

Total Nutrient Score: 4.44
Overall Rank: 890 of 8990
Fruit Rank: 15 of 20
Serving Size: 1 cup (144 g)
Calories: 408 | Carbs: 106.68 g

75% FDI for Copper
59% FDI for Iron
47% FDI for Carbohydrate
33% FDI for Vitamin B6
29% FDI for Manganese
27% FDI for Potassium
26% FDI for Fiber
26% FDI for Phosphorus
19% FDI for Thiamine (Vitamin B1)
16% FDI for Riboflavin (Vitamin B2)
15% FDI for Niacin (Vitamin B3)
14% FDI for Magnesium
12% FDI for Calcium
9% FDI for Zinc
8% FDI for Vitamin C
6% FDI for Vitamin K1
6% FDI for Protein
4% FDI for Folate
4% FDI for Vitamin A
3% FDI for Choline
3% FDI for Fats - Polyunsaturated
2% FDI for Selenium
1% FDI for Pantothenic Acid (Vitamin B5)
1% FDI for Beta-Carotene
1% FDI for Vitamin E

#16 Papayas

Total Nutrient Score: 4.36
Overall Rank: 951 of 8990
Fruit Rank: 16 of 20
Serving Size: 1 cup 1" pieces (145 g)
Calories: 62 | Carbs: 15.69 g

163% FDI for Beta-Cryptoxanthin
98% FDI for Vitamin C
46% FDI for Vitamin A
27% FDI for Lycopene
14% FDI for Folate
8% FDI for Beta-Carotene
7% FDI for Copper
7% FDI for Magnesium
7% FDI for Carbohydrate
7% FDI for Fiber
6% FDI for Potassium
6% FDI for Pantothenic Acid (Vitamin B5)
5% FDI for Vitamin K1
5% FDI for Iron
4% FDI for Vitamin B6
3% FDI for Niacin (Vitamin B3)
3% FDI for Lutein+Zeaxanthin
3% FDI for Riboflavin (Vitamin B2)
3% FDI for Vitamin E
3% FDI for Calcium
3% FDI for Thiamine (Vitamin B1)
3% FDI for Manganese
2% FDI for Phosphorus
2% FDI for Selenium
2% FDI for Choline
1% FDI for Protein
1% FDI for Zinc
1% FDI for Fats - Polyunsaturated

#17 Pears (dried)

Total Nutrient Score: 4.31
Overall Rank: 994 of 8990
Fruit Rank: 17 of 20
Serving Size: 1 cup, halves (180 g)
Calories: 472 | Carbs: 125.46 g

74% FDI for Copper
56% FDI for Carbohydrate
47% FDI for Iron
46% FDI for Vitamin K1
36% FDI for Fiber
26% FDI for Manganese
20% FDI for Potassium
20% FDI for Riboflavin (Vitamin B2)
15% FDI for Niacin (Vitamin B3)
15% FDI for Phosphorus
14% FDI for Magnesium
14% FDI for Vitamin C
10% FDI for Vitamin B6
8% FDI for Choline
6% FDI for Zinc
6% FDI for Calcium
6% FDI for Pantothenic Acid (Vitamin B5)
3% FDI for Protein
3% FDI for Fats - Polyunsaturated
2% FDI for Lutein+Zeaxanthin
1% FDI for Thiamine (Vitamin B1)

#18 Mamey Sapote

Total Nutrient Score: 4.06
Overall Rank: 1275 of 8990
Fruit Rank: 18 of 20
Serving Size: 1 cup 1" pieces (175 g)
Calories: 217 | Carbs: 56.18 g

97% FDI for Vitamin B6
45% FDI for Vitamin C
41% FDI for Copper
25% FDI for Fiber
25% FDI for Carbohydrate
25% FDI for Vitamin E
17% FDI for Iron
17% FDI for Potassium
16% FDI for Niacin (Vitamin B3)
16% FDI for Riboflavin (Vitamin B2)
16% FDI for Manganese
14% FDI for Pantothenic Acid (Vitamin B5)
9% FDI for Lutein+Zeaxanthin
8% FDI for Vitamin A
7% FDI for Phosphorus
5% FDI for Magnesium
3% FDI for Lycopene
3% FDI for Calcium
3% FDI for Zinc
3% FDI for Folate
3% FDI for Beta-Carotene
3% FDI for Protein
2% FDI for Beta-Cryptoxanthin
2% FDI for Thiamine (Vitamin B1)
2% FDI for Fats - Polyunsaturated
1% FDI for Fats - Saturated

#19 Tangerines

Total Nutrient Score: 3.99
Overall Rank: 1378 of 8990
Fruit Rank: 19 of 20
Serving Size: 1 cup, sections (195 g)
Calories: 103 | Carbs: 26.01 g

151% FDI for Beta-Cryptoxanthin
58% FDI for Vitamin C
44% FDI for Vitamin A
13% FDI for Alpha-Carotene
12% FDI for Vitamin B6
12% FDI for Carbohydrate
9% FDI for Thiamine (Vitamin B1)
9% FDI for Fiber
9% FDI for Copper
8% FDI for Pantothenic Acid (Vitamin B5)
8% FDI for Folate
7% FDI for Calcium
7% FDI for Potassium
6% FDI for Lutein+Zeaxanthin
6% FDI for Beta-Carotene
6% FDI for Phosphorus
5% FDI for Magnesium
5% FDI for Riboflavin (Vitamin B2)
5% FDI for Niacin (Vitamin B3)
4% FDI for Iron
4% FDI for Choline
3% FDI for Manganese
3% FDI for Vitamin E
2% FDI for Protein
1% FDI for Zinc
1% FDI for Fats - Polyunsaturated

#20 Figs (dried)

Total Nutrient Score: 3.98
Overall Rank: 1395 of 8990
Fruit Rank: 20 of 20
Serving Size: 1 cup (149 g)
Calories: 371 | Carbs: 95.17 g

48% FDI for Copper
42% FDI for Carbohydrate
38% FDI for Fiber
38% FDI for Iron
33% FDI for Manganese
29% FDI for Vitamin K1
24% FDI for Calcium
24% FDI for Magnesium
22% FDI for Potassium
14% FDI for Phosphorus
13% FDI for Pantothenic Acid (Vitamin B5)
12% FDI for Vitamin B6
11% FDI for Thiamine (Vitamin B1)
9% FDI for Riboflavin (Vitamin B2)
7% FDI for Zinc
6% FDI for Niacin (Vitamin B3)
5% FDI for Fats - Polyunsaturated
5% FDI for Protein
4% FDI for Choline
3% FDI for Vitamin E
3% FDI for Folate
2% FDI for Vitamin C
2% FDI for Selenium
1% FDI for Lutein+Zeaxanthin

NUTS AND SEEDS

Nutrients per One Serving

#1 Sesame Seeds

Total Nutrient Score: 24.65
Overall Rank: 16 of 8990
Nuts and Seeds Rank: 1 of 20
Serving Size: 1 cup (144 g)
Cooking preparation: whole (dried)
Calories: 825 | Carbs: 33.77 g

653% FDI for Copper
314% FDI for Fats - Polyunsaturated
262% FDI for Iron
154% FDI for Manganese
140% FDI for Calcium
129% FDI for Phosphorus
120% FDI for Magnesium
101% FDI for Zinc
95% FDI for Thiamine (Vitamin B1)
90% FDI for Selenium
88% FDI for Vitamin B6
68% FDI for Fats - Monounsaturated
45% FDI for Fiber
41% FDI for Niacin (Vitamin B3)
37% FDI for Fats - Saturated
35% FDI for Folate
27% FDI for Riboflavin (Vitamin B2)
26% FDI for Protein
15% FDI for Carbohydrate
14% FDI for Potassium
7% FDI for Choline
2% FDI for Vitamin E
1% FDI for Pantothenic Acid (Vitamin B5)

#2 Sunflower Seeds

Total Nutrient Score: 21.88
Overall Rank: 22 of 8990
Nuts and Seeds Rank: 2 of 20
Serving Size: 1 cup (128 g)
Cooking preparation: dry roasted, without salt
Calories: 745 | Carbs: 30.81 g

421% FDI for Fats - Polyunsaturated
260% FDI for Copper
223% FDI for Vitamin E
211% FDI for Phosphorus
185% FDI for Selenium
180% FDI for Pantothenic Acid (Vitamin B5)
117% FDI for Manganese
79% FDI for Vitamin B6
76% FDI for Folate
62% FDI for Zinc
61% FDI for Iron
56% FDI for Niacin (Vitamin B3)
39% FDI for Magnesium
37% FDI for Fiber
30% FDI for Fats - Monounsaturated
25% FDI for Fats - Saturated
25% FDI for Protein
24% FDI for Riboflavin (Vitamin B2)
23% FDI for Potassium
14% FDI for Carbohydrate
13% FDI for Choline
11% FDI for Thiamine (Vitamin B1)
9% FDI for Calcium
4% FDI for Vitamin K1
2% FDI for Vitamin C

#3 Brazil Nuts

Total Nutrient Score: 21.32
Overall Rank: 23 of 8990
Nuts and Seeds Rank: 3 of 20
Serving Size: 1 cup, whole (133 g)
Cooking preparation: dried, unblanched
Calories: 876 | Carbs: 15.61 g

4636% FDI for Selenium *UL used for ranking analysis
325% FDI for Fats - Polyunsaturated
258% FDI for Copper
138% FDI for Phosphorus
119% FDI for Magnesium
79% FDI for Fats - Saturated
79% FDI for Fats - Monounsaturated
71% FDI for Manganese
68% FDI for Thiamine (Vitamin B1)
50% FDI for Vitamin E
49% FDI for Zinc
40% FDI for Iron
26% FDI for Fiber
21% FDI for Calcium
19% FDI for Protein
19% FDI for Potassium
10% FDI for Vitamin B6
7% FDI for Folate
7% FDI for Choline
7% FDI for Carbohydrate
5% FDI for Pantothenic Acid (Vitamin B5)
4% FDI for Riboflavin (Vitamin B2)
2% FDI for Niacin (Vitamin B3)
1% FDI for Vitamin C

#4 Pine Nuts

Total Nutrient Score: 19.72
Overall Rank: 30 of 8990
Nuts and Seeds Rank: 4 of 20
Serving Size: 1 cup (135 g)
Cooking preparation: dried
Calories: 909 | Carbs: 17.66 g

517% FDI for Manganese *UL used for ranking analysis
460% FDI for Fats - Polyunsaturated
199% FDI for Copper
111% FDI for Phosphorus
93% FDI for Iron
91% FDI for Vitamin K1
84% FDI for Vitamin E
81% FDI for Magnesium
79% FDI for Zinc
63% FDI for Fats - Monounsaturated
41% FDI for Thiamine (Vitamin B1)
37% FDI for Niacin (Vitamin B3)
24% FDI for Fats - Saturated
24% FDI for Riboflavin (Vitamin B2)
18% FDI for Protein
17% FDI for Potassium
14% FDI for Choline
13% FDI for Fiber
12% FDI for Folate
10% FDI for Vitamin B6
8% FDI for Pantothenic Acid (Vitamin B5)
8% FDI for Carbohydrate
2% FDI for Calcium
2% FDI for Selenium
1% FDI for Vitamin A
1% FDI for Vitamin C

#5 Pumpkin and Squash Seeds

Total Nutrient Score: 17.59
Overall Rank: 39 of 8990
Nuts and Seeds Rank: 5 of 20
Serving Size: 1 cup (129 g)
Cooking preparation: dried
Calories: 721 | Carbs: 13.82 g

271% FDI for Fats - Polyunsaturated
255% FDI for Manganese
227% FDI for Phosphorus
192% FDI for Copper
182% FDI for Magnesium
142% FDI for Iron
92% FDI for Zinc
52% FDI for Fats - Monounsaturated
41% FDI for Fats - Saturated
40% FDI for Niacin (Vitamin B3)
39% FDI for Protein
29% FDI for Thiamine (Vitamin B1)
22% FDI for Potassium
22% FDI for Selenium
20% FDI for Fiber
19% FDI for Pantothenic Acid (Vitamin B5)
19% FDI for Folate
19% FDI for Vitamin E
15% FDI for Riboflavin (Vitamin B2)
15% FDI for Choline
14% FDI for Vitamin B6
12% FDI for Vitamin K1
6% FDI for Carbohydrate
6% FDI for Calcium
3% FDI for Vitamin C
2% FDI for Lutein+Zeaxanthin

#6 Cottonseed

Total Nutrient Score: 17.16
Overall Rank: 42 of 8990
Nuts and Seeds Rank: 6 of 20
Serving Size: 1 cup (149 g)
Cooking preparation: roasted (glandless)
Calories: 754 | Carbs: 32.63 g

269% FDI for Fats - Polyunsaturated
199% FDI for Copper
170% FDI for Phosphorus
156% FDI for Magnesium
141% FDI for Manganese
101% FDI for Iron
93% FDI for Thiamine (Vitamin B1)
90% FDI for Vitamin B6
87% FDI for Folate
81% FDI for Zinc
54% FDI for Fats - Saturated
49% FDI for Protein
43% FDI for Potassium
29% FDI for Riboflavin (Vitamin B2)
28% FDI for Niacin (Vitamin B3)
26% FDI for Fats - Monounsaturated
22% FDI for Vitamin A
22% FDI for Fiber
15% FDI for Calcium
15% FDI for Vitamin C
15% FDI for Carbohydrate
14% FDI for Pantothenic Acid (Vitamin B5)

#7 Almonds

Total Nutrient Score: 16.62
Overall Rank: 44 of 8990
Nuts and Seeds Rank: 7 of 20
Serving Size: 1 cup whole kernels (157 g)
Cooking preparation: oil roasted, without salt added
Calories: 953 | Carbs: 27.76 g

272% FDI for Vitamin E
212% FDI for Fats - Polyunsaturated
168% FDI for Manganese
167% FDI for Copper
137% FDI for Fats - Monounsaturated
105% FDI for Phosphorus
102% FDI for Magnesium
94% FDI for Riboflavin (Vitamin B2)
72% FDI for Iron
46% FDI for Calcium
44% FDI for Zinc
43% FDI for Fiber
36% FDI for Niacin (Vitamin B3)
33% FDI for Protein
24% FDI for Fats - Saturated
23% FDI for Potassium
15% FDI for Choline
14% FDI for Vitamin B6
12% FDI for Carbohydrate
12% FDI for Thiamine (Vitamin B1)
12% FDI for Selenium
11% FDI for Folate
7% FDI for Pantothenic Acid (Vitamin B5)

#8 Butternuts (dried)

Total Nutrient Score: 14.52
Overall Rank: 54 of 8990
Nuts and Seeds Rank: 8 of 20
Serving Size: 1 cup (120 g)
Calories: 734 | Carbs: 14.46 g

513% FDI for Fats - Polyunsaturated
342% FDI for Manganese
76% FDI for Phosphorus
68% FDI for Magnesium
60% FDI for Iron
60% FDI for Copper
52% FDI for Vitamin B6
38% FDI for Thiamine (Vitamin B1)
37% FDI for Selenium
34% FDI for Zinc
31% FDI for Fats - Monounsaturated
30% FDI for Protein
20% FDI for Folate
15% FDI for Pantothenic Acid (Vitamin B5)
15% FDI for Fiber
14% FDI for Riboflavin (Vitamin B2)
11% FDI for Potassium
8% FDI for Niacin (Vitamin B3)
6% FDI for Carbohydrate
6% FDI for Calcium
6% FDI for Fats - Saturated
5% FDI for Vitamin A
4% FDI for Vitamin C

#9 Walnuts, Black or White (dried)

Total Nutrient Score: 14.40
Overall Rank: 55 of 8990
Nuts and Seeds Rank: 9 of 20
Serving Size: 1 cup, chopped (125 g)
Calories: 774 | Carbs: 11.98 g

455% FDI for Fats - Polyunsaturated
212% FDI for Manganese
189% FDI for Copper
92% FDI for Phosphorus
60% FDI for Magnesium
56% FDI for Vitamin B6
49% FDI for Iron
48% FDI for Fats - Monounsaturated
42% FDI for Pantothenic Acid (Vitamin B5)
39% FDI for Selenium
38% FDI for Zinc
30% FDI for Protein
22% FDI for Fiber
17% FDI for Vitamin E
16% FDI for Fats - Saturated
14% FDI for Potassium
12% FDI for Riboflavin (Vitamin B2)
10% FDI for Folate
8% FDI for Calcium
7% FDI for Choline
6% FDI for Thiamine (Vitamin B1)
5% FDI for Carbohydrate
4% FDI for Vitamin K1
4% FDI for Niacin (Vitamin B3)
2% FDI for Vitamin C
2% FDI for Vitamin A

#10 Hazelnuts or Filberts

Total Nutrient Score: 13.91
Overall Rank: 61 of 8990
Nuts and Seeds Rank: 10 of 20
Serving Size: 1 cup, chopped (115 g)
Calories: 722 | Carbs: 19.2 g

309% FDI for Manganese
220% FDI for Copper
131% FDI for Fats - Monounsaturated
115% FDI for Vitamin E
91% FDI for Fats - Polyunsaturated
68% FDI for Iron
62% FDI for Thiamine (Vitamin B1)
50% FDI for Vitamin B6
48% FDI for Phosphorus
45% FDI for Magnesium
33% FDI for Folate
29% FDI for Fiber
26% FDI for Zinc
21% FDI for Pantothenic Acid (Vitamin B5)
20% FDI for Vitamin K1
19% FDI for Fats - Saturated
17% FDI for Protein
17% FDI for Potassium
13% FDI for Calcium
13% FDI for Niacin (Vitamin B3)
10% FDI for Riboflavin (Vitamin B2)
10% FDI for Choline
9% FDI for Carbohydrate
8% FDI for Vitamin C
5% FDI for Selenium
3% FDI for Lutein+Zeaxanthin

#11 Cashews (dry roasted)

Total Nutrient Score: 13.15
Overall Rank: 67 of 8990
Nuts and Seeds Rank: 11 of 20
Serving Size: 1 cup, halves and whole (137 g)
Calories: 786 | Carbs: 44.79 g

338% FDI for Copper
107% FDI for Fats - Polyunsaturated
103% FDI for Iron
96% FDI for Phosphorus
94% FDI for Fats - Monounsaturated
85% FDI for Magnesium
70% FDI for Zinc
59% FDI for Vitamin K1
49% FDI for Manganese
46% FDI for Fats - Saturated
33% FDI for Pantothenic Acid (Vitamin B5)
29% FDI for Selenium
27% FDI for Vitamin B6
24% FDI for Folate
23% FDI for Thiamine (Vitamin B1)
21% FDI for Riboflavin (Vitamin B2)
21% FDI for Protein
20% FDI for Carbohydrate
16% FDI for Potassium
15% FDI for Choline
12% FDI for Niacin (Vitamin B3)
11% FDI for Fiber
8% FDI for Vitamin E
6% FDI for Calcium

#12 Pistachios

Total Nutrient Score: 13.02
Overall Rank: 68 of 8990
Nuts and Seeds Rank: 12 of 20
Serving Size: 1 cup (123 g)
Calories: 689 | Carbs: 33.42 g

178% FDI for Copper
177% FDI for Fats - Polyunsaturated
161% FDI for Vitamin B6
89% FDI for Thiamine (Vitamin B1)
86% FDI for Phosphorus
85% FDI for Lutein+Zeaxanthin
72% FDI for Fats - Monounsaturated
64% FDI for Manganese
60% FDI for Iron
35% FDI for Magnesium
34% FDI for Fiber
27% FDI for Fats - Saturated
27% FDI for Potassium
25% FDI for Protein
25% FDI for Zinc
23% FDI for Vitamin E
21% FDI for Vitamin A
16% FDI for Folate
16% FDI for Selenium
15% FDI for Riboflavin (Vitamin B2)
15% FDI for Carbohydrate
13% FDI for Calcium
13% FDI for Pantothenic Acid (Vitamin B5)
10% FDI for Niacin (Vitamin B3)
8% FDI for Vitamin C
8% FDI for Beta-Carotene

#13 Breadnut Tree Seeds (dried)

Total Nutrient Score: 12.28
Overall Rank: 76 of 8990
Nuts and Seeds Rank: 13 of 20
Serving Size: 1 cup (160 g)
Calories: 587 | Carbs: 127.02 g

436% FDI for Copper
92% FDI for Iron
84% FDI for Vitamin B6
83% FDI for Vitamin C
68% FDI for Potassium
63% FDI for Fiber
60% FDI for Pantothenic Acid (Vitamin B5)
56% FDI for Carbohydrate
45% FDI for Folate
44% FDI for Magnesium
41% FDI for Phosphorus
28% FDI for Zinc
21% FDI for Manganese
21% FDI for Niacin (Vitamin B3)
17% FDI for Riboflavin (Vitamin B2)
15% FDI for Calcium
14% FDI for Fats - Polyunsaturated
14% FDI for Protein
12% FDI for Vitamin A
5% FDI for Selenium
4% FDI for Thiamine (Vitamin B1)
3% FDI for Fats - Saturated

#14 Chestnuts (dried)

Total Nutrient Score: 11.95
Overall Rank: 80 of 8990
Nuts and Seeds Rank: 14 of 20
Serving Size: 1 cup (155 g)
Calories: 558 | Carbs: 126.22 g

250% FDI for Manganese
226% FDI for Copper
106% FDI for Vitamin C
104% FDI for Thiamine (Vitamin B1)
79% FDI for Vitamin B6
66% FDI for Iron
56% FDI for Carbohydrate
45% FDI for Riboflavin (Vitamin B2)
42% FDI for Magnesium
42% FDI for Folate
37% FDI for Phosphorus
36% FDI for Zinc
34% FDI for Niacin (Vitamin B3)
25% FDI for Potassium
15% FDI for Pantothenic Acid (Vitamin B5)
11% FDI for Calcium
8% FDI for Protein
5% FDI for Fats - Polyunsaturated
4% FDI for Vitamin A
3% FDI for Fats - Monounsaturated
1% FDI for Fats - Saturated

#15 Hickory Nuts (dried)

Total Nutrient Score: 11.83
Overall Rank: 82 of 8990
Nuts and Seeds Rank: 15 of 20
Serving Size: 1 cup (120 g)
Calories: 788 | Carbs: 21.9 g

263% FDI for Fats - Polyunsaturated
241% FDI for Manganese
98% FDI for Copper
98% FDI for Fats - Monounsaturated
87% FDI for Thiamine (Vitamin B1)
58% FDI for Phosphorus
50% FDI for Magnesium
47% FDI for Zinc
42% FDI for Pantothenic Acid (Vitamin B5)
32% FDI for Iron
31% FDI for Fats - Saturated
20% FDI for Fiber
18% FDI for Vitamin B6
18% FDI for Selenium
15% FDI for Protein
12% FDI for Riboflavin (Vitamin B2)
12% FDI for Folate
11% FDI for Potassium
10% FDI for Carbohydrate
7% FDI for Calcium
7% FDI for Niacin (Vitamin B3)
5% FDI for Vitamin A
3% FDI for Vitamin C

#16 Watermelon Seeds (dried)

Total Nutrient Score: 11.11
Overall Rank: 95 of 8990
Nuts and Seeds Rank: 16 of 20
Serving Size: 1 cup (108 g)
Calories: 602 | Carbs: 16.53 g

303% FDI for Fats - Polyunsaturated
132% FDI for Magnesium
116% FDI for Phosphorus
101% FDI for Zinc
98% FDI for Iron
82% FDI for Copper
76% FDI for Manganese
39% FDI for Fats - Saturated
31% FDI for Protein
24% FDI for Niacin (Vitamin B3)
20% FDI for Fats - Monounsaturated
17% FDI for Thiamine (Vitamin B1)
16% FDI for Folate
15% FDI for Potassium
12% FDI for Riboflavin (Vitamin B2)
7% FDI for Pantothenic Acid (Vitamin B5)
7% FDI for Vitamin B6
7% FDI for Carbohydrate
6% FDI for Calcium

#17 Pecans

Total Nutrient Score: 11.04
Overall Rank: 97 of 8990
Nuts and Seeds Rank: 17 of 20
Serving Size: 1 cup, chopped (109 g)
Calories: 753 | Carbs: 15.11 g

236% FDI for Fats - Polyunsaturated
213% FDI for Manganese
145% FDI for Copper
111% FDI for Fats - Monounsaturated
60% FDI for Thiamine (Vitamin B1)
45% FDI for Zinc
43% FDI for Phosphorus
35% FDI for Iron
31% FDI for Magnesium
28% FDI for Fiber
25% FDI for Fats - Saturated
19% FDI for Pantothenic Acid (Vitamin B5)
18% FDI for Vitamin B6
11% FDI for Riboflavin (Vitamin B2)
10% FDI for Vitamin E
10% FDI for Protein
10% FDI for Potassium
8% FDI for Choline
8% FDI for Niacin (Vitamin B3)
8% FDI for Calcium
7% FDI for Selenium
7% FDI for Carbohydrate
6% FDI for Folate
5% FDI for Vitamin K1
2% FDI for Vitamin A
2% FDI for Beta-Cryptoxanthin
1% FDI for Vitamin C

#18 Macadamia Nuts

Total Nutrient Score: 10.95
Overall Rank: 98 of 8990
Nuts and Seeds Rank: 18 of 20
Serving Size: 1 cup, whole or halves (134 g)
Calories: 962 | Carbs: 18.52 g

241% FDI for Manganese
197% FDI for Fats - Monounsaturated
133% FDI for Thiamine (Vitamin B1)
113% FDI for Copper
62% FDI for Iron
60% FDI for Fats - Saturated
41% FDI for Magnesium
36% FDI for Phosphorus
30% FDI for Fiber
28% FDI for Vitamin B6
21% FDI for Niacin (Vitamin B3)
20% FDI for Pantothenic Acid (Vitamin B5)
20% FDI for Fats - Polyunsaturated
17% FDI for Riboflavin (Vitamin B2)
16% FDI for Zinc
11% FDI for Calcium
11% FDI for Protein
10% FDI for Potassium
9% FDI for Selenium
8% FDI for Carbohydrate
5% FDI for Vitamin E
4% FDI for Folate
2% FDI for Vitamin C

#19 Pili Nuts (dried)

Total Nutrient Score: 10.52
Overall Rank: 109 of 8990
Nuts and Seeds Rank: 19 of 20
Serving Size: 1 cup (120 g)
Calories: 863 | Carbs: 4.78 g

139% FDI for Fats - Saturated
128% FDI for Copper
121% FDI for Manganese
112% FDI for Fats - Monounsaturated
99% FDI for Phosphorus
91% FDI for Thiamine (Vitamin B1)
91% FDI for Fats - Polyunsaturated
86% FDI for Magnesium
53% FDI for Iron
32% FDI for Zinc
18% FDI for Folate
17% FDI for Calcium
13% FDI for Protein
13% FDI for Potassium
12% FDI for Pantothenic Acid (Vitamin B5)
11% FDI for Vitamin B6
9% FDI for Riboflavin (Vitamin B2)
4% FDI for Niacin (Vitamin B3)
2% FDI for Carbohydrate
2% FDI for Vitamin A

#20 Coconut Milk

Total Nutrient Score: 6.10
Overall Rank: 366 of 8990
Nuts and Seeds Rank: 20 of 20
Serving Size: 1 cup (240 g)
Calories: 552 | Carbs: 13.3 g

188% FDI for Fats - Saturated
96% FDI for Manganese
71% FDI for Copper
49% FDI for Iron
34% FDI for Phosphorus
27% FDI for Selenium
21% FDI for Magnesium
15% FDI for Zinc
14% FDI for Fiber
13% FDI for Potassium
11% FDI for Niacin (Vitamin B3)
10% FDI for Folate
9% FDI for Pantothenic Acid (Vitamin B5)
7% FDI for Vitamin C
6% FDI for Fats - Polyunsaturated
6% FDI for Fats - Monounsaturated
6% FDI for Vitamin B6
6% FDI for Carbohydrate
6% FDI for Protein
5% FDI for Thiamine (Vitamin B1)
4% FDI for Calcium
4% FDI for Choline
2% FDI for Vitamin E

SPICES AND HERBS

Nutrients per One Serving

#1 Paprika

Total Nutrient Score: 1.24
Overall Rank: 3756 of 8990
Spices and Herbs Rank: 1 of 20
Serving Size: 1 tsp (2.3 g)
Calories: 6 | Carbs: 1.24 g

38% FDI for Vitamin A
27% FDI for Beta-Cryptoxanthin
12% FDI for Beta-Carotene
10% FDI for Lutein+Zeaxanthin
6% FDI for Iron
4% FDI for Vitamin E
4% FDI for Vitamin B6
2% FDI for Vitamin K1
2% FDI for Riboflavin (Vitamin B2)
2% FDI for Fiber
2% FDI for Fats - Polyunsaturated
2% FDI for Copper
2% FDI for Manganese
1% FDI for Niacin (Vitamin B3)
1% FDI for Pantothenic Acid (Vitamin B5)
1% FDI for Potassium
1% FDI for Phosphorus

#2 Chili Powder

Total Nutrient Score: 1.00
Overall Rank: 4219 of 8990
Spices and Herbs Rank: 2 of 20
Serving Size: 1 tsp (2.7 g)
Calories: 8 | Carbs: 1.34 g

27% FDI for Vitamin A
18% FDI for Beta-Cryptoxanthin
8% FDI for Beta-Carotene
7% FDI for Vitamin E
6% FDI for Iron
4% FDI for Vitamin B6
4% FDI for Alpha-Carotene
4% FDI for Vitamin K1
3% FDI for Copper
2% FDI for Fiber
2% FDI for Fats - Polyunsaturated
2% FDI for Manganese
2% FDI for Niacin (Vitamin B3)
2% FDI for Riboflavin (Vitamin B2)
1% FDI for Phosphorus
1% FDI for Potassium
1% FDI for Selenium
1% FDI for Zinc

#3 Cayenne or Red Pepper

Total Nutrient Score: 0.85
Overall Rank: 4500 of 8990
Spices and Herbs Rank: 3 of 20
Serving Size: 1 tsp (1.8 g)
Calories: 6 | Carbs: 1.02 g

25% FDI for Vitamin A
22% FDI for Beta-Cryptoxanthin
8% FDI for Beta-Carotene
6% FDI for Lutein+Zeaxanthin
4% FDI for Vitamin E
3% FDI for Vitamin B6
2% FDI for Iron
2% FDI for Vitamin K1
2% FDI for Manganese
2% FDI for Vitamin C
2% FDI for Fats - Polyunsaturated
1% FDI for Fiber
1% FDI for Riboflavin (Vitamin B2)

#4 Cloves (ground)

Total Nutrient Score: 0.74
Overall Rank: 4651 of 8990
Spices and Herbs Rank: 4 of 20
Serving Size: 1 tsp (2.1 g)
Calories: 6 | Carbs: 1.38 g

55% FDI for Manganese
4% FDI for Vitamin K1
3% FDI for Iron
2% FDI for Fiber
1% FDI for Calcium
1% FDI for Vitamin E
1% FDI for Magnesium

#5 Turmeric (ground)

Total Nutrient Score: 0.64
Overall Rank: 4802 of 8990
Spices and Herbs Rank: 5 of 20
Serving Size: 1 tsp (3 g)
Calories: 9 | Carbs: 2.01 g

26% FDI for Manganese
21% FDI for Iron
4% FDI for Copper
2% FDI for Fiber
1% FDI for Magnesium
1% FDI for Potassium
1% FDI for Phosphorus
1% FDI for Zinc

#6 Thyme (dried)

Total Nutrient Score: 0.52
Overall Rank: 4951 of 8990
Spices and Herbs Rank: 6 of 20
Serving Size: 1 tsp, leaves (1 g)
Calories: 3 | Carbs: 0.64 g

21% FDI for Vitamin K1
16% FDI for Iron
3% FDI for Manganese
2% FDI for Calcium
1% FDI for Vitamin A
1% FDI for Fiber
1% FDI for Copper

#7 Poppy Seed

Total Nutrient Score: 0.45
Overall Rank: 5038 of 8990
Spices and Herbs Rank: 7 of 20
Serving Size: 1 tsp (2.8 g)
Calories: 15 | Carbs: 0.79 g

8% FDI for Manganese
8% FDI for Fats - Polyunsaturated
5% FDI for Copper
4% FDI for Calcium
3% FDI for Phosphorus
3% FDI for Iron
2% FDI for Magnesium
2% FDI for Zinc
2% FDI for Thiamine (Vitamin B1)
1% FDI for Fiber

#8 Ginger (ground)

Total Nutrient Score: 0.41
Overall Rank: 5077 of 8990
Spices and Herbs Rank: 8 of 20
Serving Size: 1 tsp (1.8 g)
Calories: 6 | Carbs: 1.29 g

26% FDI for Manganese
5% FDI for Iron
2% FDI for Selenium
1% FDI for Niacin (Vitamin B3)
1% FDI for Copper

#9 Cumin Seed

Total Nutrient Score: 0.38
Overall Rank: 5103 of 8990
Spices and Herbs Rank: 9 of 20
Serving Size: 1 tsp, whole (2.1 g)
Calories: 8 | Carbs: 0.93 g

17% FDI for Iron
3% FDI for Manganese
2% FDI for Calcium
2% FDI for Copper
2% FDI for Magnesium
1% FDI for Phosphorus
1% FDI for Thiamine (Vitamin B1)

#10 Cardamom

Total Nutrient Score: 0.37
Overall Rank: 5106 of 8990
Spices and Herbs Rank: 10 of 20
Serving Size: 1 tsp, ground (2 g)
Calories: 6 | Carbs: 1.37 g

24% FDI for Manganese
4% FDI for Iron
2% FDI for Fiber
1% FDI for Zinc
1% FDI for Magnesium

#11 Fenugreek Seed

Total Nutrient Score: 0.37
Overall Rank: 5108 of 8990
Spices and Herbs Rank: 11 of 20
Serving Size: 1 tsp (3.7 g)
Calories: 12 | Carbs: 2.16 g

16% FDI for Iron
5% FDI for Copper
2% FDI for Fiber
2% FDI for Manganese
2% FDI for Vitamin B6
2% FDI for Magnesium
2% FDI for Phosphorus
1% FDI for Riboflavin (Vitamin B2)
1% FDI for Thiamine (Vitamin B1)

#12 Celery Seed

Total Nutrient Score: 0.37
Overall Rank: 5110 of 8990
Spices and Herbs Rank: 12 of 20
Serving Size: 1 tsp (2 g)
Calories: 8 | Carbs: 0.83 g

11% FDI for Iron
7% FDI for Manganese
4% FDI for Calcium
3% FDI for Copper
2% FDI for Magnesium
2% FDI for Phosphorus
1% FDI for Vitamin B6
1% FDI for Zinc

#13 Cinnamon (ground)

Total Nutrient Score: 0.36
Overall Rank: 5119 of 8990
Spices and Herbs Rank: 13 of 20
Serving Size: 1 tsp (2.6 g)
Calories: 6 | Carbs: 2.1 g

20% FDI for Manganese
4% FDI for Fiber
3% FDI for Iron
3% FDI for Calcium
1% FDI for Vitamin K1
1% FDI for Copper

#14 Basil (dried or fresh)

Total Nutrient Score: 0.36
Overall Rank: 5120 of 8990
Spices and Herbs Rank: 14 of 20
Serving Size: 1 tsp, leaves (0.7 g)
Calories: 2 | Carbs: 0.33 g

15% FDI for Vitamin K1
8% FDI for Iron
3% FDI for Manganese
2% FDI for Copper
2% FDI for Calcium
1% FDI for Magnesium

#15 Curry Powder

Total Nutrient Score: 0.33
Overall Rank: 5139 of 8990
Spices and Herbs Rank: 15 of 20
Serving Size: 1 tsp (2 g)
Calories: 6 | Carbs: 1.12 g

7% FDI for Manganese
5% FDI for Iron
3% FDI for Vitamin E
3% FDI for Fiber
3% FDI for Copper
3% FDI for Vitamin K1
1% FDI for Selenium
1% FDI for Magnesium
1% FDI for Calcium
1% FDI for Phosphorus

#16 Black Pepper

Total Nutrient Score: 0.33
Overall Rank: 5141 of 8990
Spices and Herbs Rank: 16 of 20
Serving Size: 1 tsp, ground (2.3 g)
Calories: 6 | Carbs: 1.47 g

13% FDI for Manganese
5% FDI for Vitamin K1
3% FDI for Copper
3% FDI for Iron
2% FDI for Fiber
1% FDI for Calcium

#17 Mustard Seed (ground)

Total Nutrient Score: 0.30
Overall Rank: 5157 of 8990
Spices and Herbs Rank: 17 of 20
Serving Size: 1 tsp (2 g)
Calories: 10 | Carbs: 0.56 g

8% FDI for Selenium
3% FDI for Fats - Polyunsaturated
2% FDI for Phosphorus
2% FDI for Iron
2% FDI for Manganese
2% FDI for Magnesium
1% FDI for Copper
1% FDI for Thiamine (Vitamin B1)
1% FDI for Fats - Monounsaturated
1% FDI for Zinc

#18 Coriander Leaf (dried)

Total Nutrient Score: 0.29
Overall Rank: 5166 of 8990
Spices and Herbs Rank: 18 of 20
Serving Size: 1 tsp (0.6 g)
Calories: 2 | Carbs: 0.31 g

10% FDI for Vitamin K1
4% FDI for Vitamin C
3% FDI for Iron
2% FDI for Manganese
1% FDI for Copper
1% FDI for Vitamin A

#19 Sage (ground)

Total Nutrient Score: 0.29
Overall Rank: 5167 of 8990
Spices and Herbs Rank: 19 of 20
Serving Size: 1 tsp (0.7 g)
Calories: 2 | Carbs: 0.43 g

15% FDI for Vitamin K1
3% FDI for Iron
1% FDI for Vitamin B6
1% FDI for Vitamin A
1% FDI for Calcium

#20 Fennel

Total Nutrient Score: 0.27
Overall Rank: 5181 of 8990
Spices and Herbs Rank: 20 of 20
Serving Size: 1 tsp, whole (2 g)
Calories: 7 | Carbs: 1.05 g

6% FDI for Manganese
5% FDI for Iron
2% FDI for Calcium
2% FDI for Copper
2% FDI for Fiber
2% FDI for Magnesium
1% FDI for Phosphorus

DAIRY AND EGGS

Nutrients per One Serving

#1 Egg Yolk (dried)

Total Nutrient Score: 14.99
Overall Rank: 47 of 8990
Dairy and Egg products Rank: 1 of 20
Serving Size: 1 cup, sifted (67 g)
Calories: 448 | Carbs: 0.44 g

293% FDI for Choline
170% FDI for Selenium
143% FDI for Vitamin B12
121% FDI for Pantothenic Acid (Vitamin B5)
100% FDI for Phosphorus
86% FDI for Fats - Polyunsaturated
80% FDI for Iron
77% FDI for Omega-3 (DHA, 22:6)
65% FDI for Riboflavin (Vitamin B2)
50% FDI for Fats - Saturated
47% FDI for Zinc
39% FDI for Fats - Monounsaturated
38% FDI for Vitamin B6
36% FDI for Vitamin A
35% FDI for Folate
23% FDI for Protein
22% FDI for Thiamine (Vitamin B1)
21% FDI for Vitamin E
19% FDI for Calcium
18% FDI for Lutein+Zeaxanthin
9% FDI for Beta-Cryptoxanthin
6% FDI for Vitamin D3
5% FDI for Manganese
4% FDI for Magnesium
4% FDI for Potassium
4% FDI for Alpha-Carotene
1% FDI for Vitamin K1

#2 Whole Egg (dried)

Total Nutrient Score: 14.39
Overall Rank: 56 of 8990
Dairy and Egg products Rank: 2 of 20
Serving Size: 1 cup, sifted (85 g)
Calories: 503 | Carbs: 0.96 g

255% FDI for Selenium
196% FDI for Choline
129% FDI for Riboflavin (Vitamin B2)
105% FDI for Vitamin B12
94% FDI for Pantothenic Acid (Vitamin B5)
77% FDI for Omega-3 (DHA, 22:6)
77% FDI for Iron
76% FDI for Phosphorus
71% FDI for Fats - Polyunsaturated
47% FDI for Fats - Saturated
41% FDI for Protein
36% FDI for Fats - Monounsaturated
33% FDI for Vitamin B6
28% FDI for Vitamin A
25% FDI for Folate
24% FDI for Zinc
22% FDI for Vitamin E
21% FDI for Calcium
19% FDI for Copper
17% FDI for Lutein+Zeaxanthin
13% FDI for Thiamine (Vitamin B1)
10% FDI for Potassium
7% FDI for Magnesium
6% FDI for Beta-Cryptoxanthin
6% FDI for Vitamin D3
2% FDI for Manganese
2% FDI for Niacin (Vitamin B3)
1% FDI for Vitamin K1

#3 Sweet Whey

Total Nutrient Score: 13.91
Overall Rank: 62 of 8990
Dairy and Egg products Rank: 3 of 20
Serving Size: 1 cup (145 g)
Calories: 512 | Carbs: 107.97 g

246% FDI for Riboflavin (Vitamin B2)
193% FDI for Phosphorus
163% FDI for Pantothenic Acid (Vitamin B5)
143% FDI for Vitamin B12
115% FDI for Calcium
72% FDI for Selenium
65% FDI for Vitamin B6
64% FDI for Potassium
63% FDI for Thiamine (Vitamin B1)
61% FDI for Magnesium
59% FDI for Choline
48% FDI for Carbohydrate
26% FDI for Zinc
19% FDI for Protein
16% FDI for Iron
11% FDI for Niacin (Vitamin B3)
11% FDI for Copper
4% FDI for Folate
4% FDI for Fats - Saturated
2% FDI for Vitamin C
1% FDI for Vitamin A
1% FDI for Fats - Monounsaturated

#4 Whole Milk (dried)

Total Nutrient Score: 11.04
Overall Rank: 96 of 8990
Dairy and Egg products Rank: 4 of 20
Serving Size: 1 cup (128 g)
Calories: 635 | Carbs: 49.18 g

173% FDI for Vitamin B12
142% FDI for Phosphorus
119% FDI for Riboflavin (Vitamin B2)
117% FDI for Calcium
79% FDI for Fats - Saturated
58% FDI for Pantothenic Acid (Vitamin B5)
40% FDI for Vitamin A
39% FDI for Zinc
38% FDI for Selenium
36% FDI for Potassium
34% FDI for Protein
30% FDI for Thiamine (Vitamin B1)
30% FDI for Vitamin B6
27% FDI for Choline
26% FDI for Magnesium
25% FDI for Fats - Monounsaturated
22% FDI for Carbohydrate
12% FDI for Vitamin C
12% FDI for Folate
11% FDI for Copper
9% FDI for Fats - Polyunsaturated
8% FDI for Iron
5% FDI for Niacin (Vitamin B3)
5% FDI for Vitamin E
4% FDI for Vitamin K1
2% FDI for Manganese
1% FDI for Beta-Carotene

#5 Swiss Cheese

Total Nutrient Score: 8.25
Overall Rank: 172 of 8990
Dairy and Egg products Rank: 5 of 20
Serving Size: 1 cup, diced (132 g)
Calories: 519 | Carbs: 1.9 g

168% FDI for Vitamin B12
118% FDI for Calcium
108% FDI for Phosphorus
89% FDI for Fats - Saturated
72% FDI for Selenium
52% FDI for Zinc
46% FDI for Vitamin A
36% FDI for Protein
31% FDI for Riboflavin (Vitamin B2)
27% FDI for Fats - Monounsaturated
18% FDI for Fats - Polyunsaturated
10% FDI for Magnesium
9% FDI for Pantothenic Acid (Vitamin B5)
7% FDI for Vitamin B6
7% FDI for Copper
5% FDI for Vitamin E
4% FDI for Choline
3% FDI for Folate
2% FDI for Vitamin K1
2% FDI for Iron
2% FDI for Potassium
2% FDI for Beta-Carotene
1% FDI for Manganese
1% FDI for Vitamin K2 M-4
1% FDI for Thiamine (Vitamin B1)

#6 Feta Cheese

Total Nutrient Score: 7.41
Overall Rank: 215 of 8990
Dairy and Egg products Rank: 6 of 20
Serving Size: 1 cup, crumbled (150 g)
Calories: 396 | Carbs: 6.14 g

106% FDI for Vitamin B12
97% FDI for Riboflavin (Vitamin B2)
83% FDI for Fats - Saturated
74% FDI for Calcium
72% FDI for Phosphorus
49% FDI for Vitamin B6
41% FDI for Selenium
39% FDI for Zinc
29% FDI for Pantothenic Acid (Vitamin B5)
21% FDI for Protein
21% FDI for Vitamin A
19% FDI for Thiamine (Vitamin B1)
17% FDI for Fats - Monounsaturated
12% FDI for Iron
12% FDI for Folate
11% FDI for Fats - Polyunsaturated
9% FDI for Niacin (Vitamin B3)
7% FDI for Magnesium
5% FDI for Copper
4% FDI for Choline
3% FDI for Vitamin K1
3% FDI for Carbohydrate
2% FDI for Potassium
2% FDI for Manganese
2% FDI for Vitamin E

#7 Cheddar Cheese

Total Nutrient Score: 6.98
Overall Rank: 262 of 8990
Dairy and Egg products Rank: 7 of 20
Serving Size: 1 cup, diced (132 g)
Calories: 533 | Carbs: 4.08 g

94% FDI for Calcium
92% FDI for Fats - Saturated
86% FDI for Phosphorus
68% FDI for Selenium
60% FDI for Vitamin B12
55% FDI for Vitamin A
44% FDI for Zinc
43% FDI for Riboflavin (Vitamin B2)
31% FDI for Fats - Monounsaturated
30% FDI for Protein
19% FDI for Fats - Polyunsaturated
11% FDI for Pantothenic Acid (Vitamin B5)
9% FDI for Folate
9% FDI for Magnesium
7% FDI for Vitamin B6
6% FDI for Vitamin E
6% FDI for Omega-3 (EPA, 20:5)
4% FDI for Copper
4% FDI for Vitamin K1
4% FDI for Choline
3% FDI for Thiamine (Vitamin B1)
2% FDI for Iron
2% FDI for Beta-Carotene
2% FDI for Potassium
2% FDI for Vitamin K2 M-4
2% FDI for Carbohydrate
2% FDI for Manganese

#8 Acid Whey

Total Nutrient Score: 6.86
Overall Rank: 273 of 8990
Dairy and Egg products Rank: 8 of 20
Serving Size: 1 cup (57 g)
Calories: 193 | Carbs: 41.87 g

117% FDI for Calcium
110% FDI for Phosphorus
90% FDI for Riboflavin (Vitamin B2)
64% FDI for Pantothenic Acid (Vitamin B5)
59% FDI for Vitamin B12
33% FDI for Zinc
30% FDI for Thiamine (Vitamin B1)
28% FDI for Selenium
28% FDI for Potassium
27% FDI for Vitamin B6
27% FDI for Magnesium
23% FDI for Choline
19% FDI for Carbohydrate
9% FDI for Iron
7% FDI for Protein
5% FDI for Folate
4% FDI for Niacin (Vitamin B3)
3% FDI for Copper
1% FDI for Vitamin A

#9 Provolone Cheese

Total Nutrient Score: 6.36
Overall Rank: 320 of 8990
Dairy and Egg products Rank: 9 of 20
Serving Size: 1 cup, diced (132 g)
Calories: 463 | Carbs: 2.82 g

100% FDI for Calcium
94% FDI for Phosphorus
83% FDI for Fats - Saturated
80% FDI for Vitamin B12
39% FDI for Vitamin A
39% FDI for Zinc
35% FDI for Selenium
34% FDI for Protein
33% FDI for Riboflavin (Vitamin B2)
24% FDI for Fats - Monounsaturated
13% FDI for Pantothenic Acid (Vitamin B5)
10% FDI for Fats - Polyunsaturated
9% FDI for Magnesium
9% FDI for Iron
7% FDI for Vitamin B6
4% FDI for Potassium
4% FDI for Copper
4% FDI for Choline
4% FDI for Vitamin K1
3% FDI for Folate
2% FDI for Thiamine (Vitamin B1)
2% FDI for Vitamin E
2% FDI for Beta-Carotene
1% FDI for Niacin (Vitamin B3)
1% FDI for Carbohydrate

#10 American Cheese Spread

Total Nutrient Score: 6.30
Overall Rank: 324 of 8990
Dairy and Egg products Rank: 10 of 20
Serving Size: 1 cup, diced (140 g)
Calories: 406 | Carbs: 12.22 g

175% FDI for Phosphorus
79% FDI for Calcium
69% FDI for Fats - Saturated
46% FDI for Riboflavin (Vitamin B2)
33% FDI for Zinc
30% FDI for Vitamin A
29% FDI for Selenium
23% FDI for Vitamin B12
23% FDI for Protein
22% FDI for Fats - Monounsaturated
19% FDI for Pantothenic Acid (Vitamin B5)
13% FDI for Vitamin B6
10% FDI for Magnesium
9% FDI for Choline
9% FDI for Fats - Polyunsaturated
7% FDI for Potassium
6% FDI for Iron
6% FDI for Thiamine (Vitamin B1)
5% FDI for Carbohydrate
5% FDI for Copper
3% FDI for Vitamin K1
3% FDI for Folate
2% FDI for Vitamin E
2% FDI for Beta-Carotene
1% FDI for Manganese
1% FDI for Niacin (Vitamin B3)

#11 Muenster Cheese

Total Nutrient Score: 6.24
Overall Rank: 333 of 8990
Dairy and Egg products Rank: 11 of 20
Serving Size: 1 cup, diced (132 g)
Calories: 486 | Carbs: 1.48 g

95% FDI for Calcium
93% FDI for Fats - Saturated
88% FDI for Phosphorus
81% FDI for Vitamin B12
45% FDI for Vitamin A
35% FDI for Selenium
34% FDI for Zinc
32% FDI for Riboflavin (Vitamin B2)
31% FDI for Protein
29% FDI for Fats - Monounsaturated
9% FDI for Fats - Polyunsaturated
9% FDI for Magnesium
7% FDI for Iron
6% FDI for Vitamin B6
5% FDI for Pantothenic Acid (Vitamin B5)
5% FDI for Copper
4% FDI for Vitamin K1
4% FDI for Folate
4% FDI for Potassium
4% FDI for Choline
2% FDI for Vitamin E
1% FDI for Thiamine (Vitamin B1)

#12 Colby Cheese

Total Nutrient Score: 6.17
Overall Rank: 350 of 8990
Dairy and Egg products Rank: 12 of 20
Serving Size: 1 cup, diced (132 g)
Calories: 520 | Carbs: 3.39 g

99% FDI for Fats - Saturated
90% FDI for Calcium
86% FDI for Phosphorus
46% FDI for Vitamin B12
44% FDI for Vitamin A
38% FDI for Riboflavin (Vitamin B2)
37% FDI for Zinc
35% FDI for Selenium
31% FDI for Protein
31% FDI for Fats - Monounsaturated
13% FDI for Fats - Polyunsaturated
13% FDI for Iron
8% FDI for Magnesium
8% FDI for Vitamin B6
6% FDI for Copper
6% FDI for Folate
6% FDI for Pantothenic Acid (Vitamin B5)
5% FDI for Vitamin K1
4% FDI for Choline
4% FDI for Potassium
2% FDI for Vitamin E
2% FDI for Beta-Carotene
2% FDI for Thiamine (Vitamin B1)
2% FDI for Carbohydrate

#13 Brick Cheese

Total Nutrient Score: 6.14
Overall Rank: 361 of 8990
Dairy and Egg products Rank: 13 of 20
Serving Size: 1 cup, diced (132 g)
Calories: 490 | Carbs: 3.68 g

92% FDI for Fats - Saturated
89% FDI for Calcium
85% FDI for Phosphorus
69% FDI for Vitamin B12
48% FDI for Vitamin A
36% FDI for Riboflavin (Vitamin B2)
35% FDI for Selenium
31% FDI for Zinc
31% FDI for Protein
28% FDI for Fats - Monounsaturated
10% FDI for Fats - Polyunsaturated
8% FDI for Magnesium
8% FDI for Pantothenic Acid (Vitamin B5)
7% FDI for Iron
7% FDI for Vitamin B6
7% FDI for Folate
4% FDI for Vitamin K1
4% FDI for Potassium
4% FDI for Choline
4% FDI for Copper
2% FDI for Vitamin E
2% FDI for Beta-Carotene
2% FDI for Carbohydrate
2% FDI for Thiamine (Vitamin B1)

#14 Limburger Cheese

Total Nutrient Score: 6.08
Overall Rank: 367 of 8990
Dairy and Egg products Rank: 14 of 20
Serving Size: 1 cup (134 g)
Calories: 438 | Carbs: 0.66 g

83% FDI for Fats - Saturated
75% FDI for Phosphorus
67% FDI for Calcium
58% FDI for Vitamin B12
52% FDI for Riboflavin (Vitamin B2)
52% FDI for Vitamin A
35% FDI for Selenium
32% FDI for Pantothenic Acid (Vitamin B5)
29% FDI for Fats - Monounsaturated
27% FDI for Protein
26% FDI for Zinc
20% FDI for Folate
9% FDI for Thiamine (Vitamin B1)
9% FDI for Vitamin B6
7% FDI for Magnesium
7% FDI for Fats - Polyunsaturated
4% FDI for Vitamin K1
4% FDI for Choline
4% FDI for Potassium
3% FDI for Copper
2% FDI for Manganese
2% FDI for Iron
2% FDI for Vitamin E
1% FDI for Niacin (Vitamin B3)

#15 Monterey Cheese

Total Nutrient Score: 6.02
Overall Rank: 380 of 8990
Dairy and Egg products Rank: 15 of 20
Serving Size: 1 cup, diced (132 g)
Calories: 492 | Carbs: 0.9 g

99% FDI for Calcium
93% FDI for Fats – Saturated
84% FDI for Phosphorus
46% FDI for Vitamin B12
40% FDI for Riboflavin (Vitamin B2)
36% FDI for Zinc
35% FDI for Selenium
34% FDI for Vitamin A
32% FDI for Protein
29% FDI for Fats – Monounsaturated
12% FDI for Iron
12% FDI for Fats – Polyunsaturated
9% FDI for Magnesium
8% FDI for Vitamin B6
6% FDI for Folate
6% FDI for Pantothenic Acid (Vitamin B5)
5% FDI for Copper
4% FDI for Vitamin K1
4% FDI for Choline
2% FDI for Potassium
2% FDI for Vitamin E
2% FDI for Beta-Carotene
2% FDI for Thiamine (Vitamin B1)

#16 Fontina Cheese

Total Nutrient Score: 5.98
Overall Rank: 367 of 8990
Dairy and Egg products Rank: 16 of 20
Serving Size: 1 cup, diced (132 g)
Calories: 513 | Carbs: 2.05 g

94% FDI for Fats – Saturated
93% FDI for Vitamin B12
73% FDI for Calcium
65% FDI for Phosphorus
42% FDI for Zinc
40% FDI for Vitamin A
35% FDI for Selenium
34% FDI for Protein
29% FDI for Fats – Monounsaturated
22% FDI for Fats – Polyunsaturated
21% FDI for Riboflavin (Vitamin B2)
11% FDI for Pantothenic Acid (Vitamin B5)
8% FDI for Vitamin B6
4% FDI for Magnesium
4% FDI for Vitamin K1
4% FDI for Iron
4% FDI for Choline
4% FDI for Copper
2% FDI for Vitamin E
2% FDI for Thiamine (Vitamin B1)
2% FDI for Folate
2% FDI for Potassium
1% FDI for Niacin (Vitamin B3)

#17 Port De Salut Cheese

Total Nutrient Score: 5.81
Overall Rank: 419 of 8990
Dairy and Egg products Rank: 17 of 20
Serving Size: 1 cup, diced (132 g)
Calories: 465 | Carbs: 0.75 g

86% FDI for Calcium
83% FDI for Vitamin B12
82% FDI for Fats - Saturated
68% FDI for Phosphorus
48% FDI for Vitamin A
35% FDI for Selenium
31% FDI for Protein
31% FDI for Zinc
31% FDI for Fats - Monounsaturated
24% FDI for Riboflavin (Vitamin B2)
10% FDI for Fats - Polyunsaturated
8% FDI for Magnesium
7% FDI for Iron
6% FDI for Folate
6% FDI for Pantothenic Acid (Vitamin B5)
5% FDI for Vitamin B6
4% FDI for Vitamin K1
4% FDI for Potassium
4% FDI for Choline
3% FDI for Copper
2% FDI for Vitamin E
2% FDI for Thiamine (Vitamin B1)

#18 Parmesan Cheese

Total Nutrient Score: 5.73
Overall Rank: 428 of 8990
Dairy and Egg products Rank: 18 of 20
Serving Size: 1 cup (100 g)
Cooking preparation: grated
Calories: 420 | Carbs: 13.91 g

90% FDI for Phosphorus
85% FDI for Calcium
63% FDI for Selenium
58% FDI for Vitamin B12
57% FDI for Fats - Saturated
38% FDI for Zinc
32% FDI for Vitamin A
28% FDI for Protein
28% FDI for Riboflavin (Vitamin B2)
18% FDI for Fats - Monounsaturated
14% FDI for Fats - Polyunsaturated
9% FDI for Pantothenic Acid (Vitamin B5)
8% FDI for Magnesium
6% FDI for Vitamin B6
6% FDI for Carbohydrate
6% FDI for Iron
4% FDI for Copper
4% FDI for Potassium
4% FDI for Vitamin E
3% FDI for Manganese
3% FDI for Choline
2% FDI for Thiamine (Vitamin B1)
2% FDI for Vitamin K1
2% FDI for Folate
1% FDI for Beta-Carotene
1% FDI for Vitamin K2 M-4

#19 Hard Boiled Egg

Total Nutrient Score: 5.68
Overall Rank: 437 of 8990
Dairy and Egg products Rank: 20 of 20
Serving Size: 1 cup, chopped (136 g)
Cooking preparation: cooked, hard-boiled
Calories: 211 | Carbs: 1.52 g

76% FDI for Selenium
73% FDI for Choline
63% FDI for Vitamin B12
54% FDI for Riboflavin (Vitamin B2)
38% FDI for Pantothenic Acid (Vitamin B5)
33% FDI for Phosphorus
24% FDI for Omega-3 (DHA, 22:6)
24% FDI for Vitamin A
20% FDI for Iron
19% FDI for Fats - Polyunsaturated
17% FDI for Protein
16% FDI for Fats - Saturated
15% FDI for Folate
14% FDI for Fats - Monounsaturated
13% FDI for Zinc
13% FDI for Vitamin B6
11% FDI for Lutein+Zeaxanthin
9% FDI for Vitamin E
8% FDI for Thiamine (Vitamin B1)
7% FDI for Calcium
4% FDI for Potassium
3% FDI for Magnesium
3% FDI for Omega-3 (EPA, 20:5)
3% FDI for Beta-Cryptoxanthin
2% FDI for Vitamin D3
2% FDI for Copper
2% FDI for Manganese

#19 Mexican Cheese (queso anejo)

Total Nutrient Score: 5.62
Overall Rank: 444 of 8990
Dairy and Egg products Rank: 19 of 20
Serving Size: 1 cup, crumbled (132 g)
Calories: 492 | Carbs: 6.11 g

93% FDI for Fats - Saturated
90% FDI for Calcium
84% FDI for Phosphorus
76% FDI for Vitamin B12
35% FDI for Zinc
35% FDI for Selenium
28% FDI for Protein
28% FDI for Fats - Monounsaturated
21% FDI for Riboflavin (Vitamin B2)
12% FDI for Fats - Polyunsaturated
10% FDI for Vitamin A
9% FDI for Magnesium
8% FDI for Iron
7% FDI for Pantothenic Acid (Vitamin B5)
5% FDI for Vitamin B6
4% FDI for Vitamin K1
4% FDI for Choline
3% FDI for Carbohydrate
2% FDI for Potassium
2% FDI for Vitamin E
2% FDI for Thiamine (Vitamin B1)
2% FDI for Manganese
1% FDI for Copper

LEGUMES

Nutrients per One Serving

#1 Peanuts (Spanish, Virginia, Valencia)

Total Nutrient Score: 14.94
Overall Rank: 49 of 8990
Legumes Rank: 1 of 20
Serving Size: 1 cup (146 g)
Cooking preparation: raw
Calories: 832 | Carbs: 23.11 g

252% FDI for Fats - Polyunsaturated
168% FDI for Manganese
146% FDI for Copper
145% FDI for Niacin (Vitamin B3)
88% FDI for Folate
81% FDI for Fats - Monounsaturated
82% FDI for Thiamine (Vitamin B1)
81% FDI for Phosphorus
71% FDI for Iron
65% FDI for Magnesium
52% FDI for Pantothenic Acid (Vitamin B5)
39% FDI for Vitamin B6
38% FDI for Fats - Saturated
38% FDI for Protein
37% FDI for Fiber
28% FDI for Zinc
23% FDI for Potassium
19% FDI for Selenium
16% FDI for Calcium
15% FDI for Riboflavin (Vitamin B2)
10% FDI for Carbohydrate

#2 Soybeans (roasted)

Total Nutrient Score: 13.89
Overall Rank: 63 of 8990
Legumes Rank: 2 of 20
Serving Size: 1 cup (172 g)
Cooking preparation: roasted
Calories: 807 | Carbs: 51.98 g

247% FDI for Fats - Polyunsaturated
161% FDI for Manganese
158% FDI for Copper
91% FDI for Folate
89% FDI for Phosphorus
84% FDI for Iron
80% FDI for Fiber
66% FDI for Protein
60% FDI for Selenium
59% FDI for Magnesium
54% FDI for Potassium
49% FDI for Zinc
28% FDI for Vitamin B6
24% FDI for Fats - Monounsaturated
24% FDI for Calcium
23% FDI for Fats - Saturated
23% FDI for Carbohydrate
19% FDI for Riboflavin (Vitamin B2)
16% FDI for Pantothenic Acid (Vitamin B5)
15% FDI for Niacin (Vitamin B3)
14% FDI for Thiamine (Vitamin B1)
4% FDI for Vitamin C

#3 Soy Flour (full-fat, roasted)

Total Nutrient Score: 10.55
Overall Rank: 108 of 8990
Legumes Rank: 3 of 20
Serving Size: 1 cup, stirred (85 g)
Cooking preparation: roasted
Calories: 373 | Carbs: 25.82 g

210% FDI for Copper
105% FDI for Fats - Polyunsaturated
77% FDI for Manganese
76% FDI for Vitamin K1
75% FDI for Magnesium
62% FDI for Iron
62% FDI for Riboflavin (Vitamin B2)
58% FDI for Phosphorus
48% FDI for Folate
37% FDI for Potassium
32% FDI for Protein
29% FDI for Thiamine (Vitamin B1)
28% FDI for Zinc
23% FDI for Vitamin B6
22% FDI for Fiber
21% FDI for Pantothenic Acid (Vitamin B5)
17% FDI for Niacin (Vitamin B3)
16% FDI for Calcium
12% FDI for Selenium
11% FDI for Carbohydrate
11% FDI for Vitamin E
10% FDI for Fats - Monounsaturated
10% FDI for Fats - Saturated
3% FDI for Vitamin A
1% FDI for Beta-Carotene

#4 Natto

Total Nutrient Score: 10.37
Overall Rank: 113 of 8990
Legumes Rank: 4 of 20
Serving Size: 1 cup (175 g)
Calories: 369 | Carbs: 22.19 g

188% FDI for Iron
130% FDI for Copper
116% FDI for Manganese
109% FDI for Fats - Polyunsaturated
51% FDI for Vitamin K1
48% FDI for Zinc
48% FDI for Magnesium
43% FDI for Phosphorus
38% FDI for Calcium
34% FDI for Protein
28% FDI for Selenium
27% FDI for Potassium
26% FDI for Riboflavin (Vitamin B2)
25% FDI for Vitamin C
25% FDI for Fiber
23% FDI for Thiamine (Vitamin B1)
18% FDI for Choline
18% FDI for Vitamin B6
11% FDI for Fats - Monounsaturated
10% FDI for Fats - Saturated
10% FDI for Carbohydrate
8% FDI for Pantothenic Acid (Vitamin B5)
4% FDI for Folate

#5 Soybean Curd Cheese

Total Nutrient Score: 9.8590
Overall Rank: 133 of 8990
Legumes Rank: 5 of 20
Serving Size: 1 cup (225 g)
Calories: 340 | Carbs: 15.52 g

158% FDI for Iron
122% FDI for Magnesium
103% FDI for Fats - Polyunsaturated
95% FDI for Copper
87% FDI for Manganese
71% FDI for Phosphorus
69% FDI for Selenium
42% FDI for Calcium
35% FDI for Zinc
28% FDI for Protein
26% FDI for Choline
24% FDI for Riboflavin (Vitamin B2)
13% FDI for Vitamin K1
13% FDI for Folate
12% FDI for Vitamin B6
10% FDI for Fats - Monounsaturated
10% FDI for Fats - Saturated
10% FDI for Potassium
9% FDI for Vitamin E
7% FDI for Niacin (Vitamin B3)
7% FDI for Carbohydrate
5% FDI for Pantothenic Acid (Vitamin B5)
3% FDI for Vitamin A
1% FDI for Beta-Carotene

#6 Tempeh

Total Nutrient Score: 6.74
Overall Rank: 276 of 8990
Legumes Rank: 6 of 20
Serving Size: 1 cup (166 g)
Calories: 319 | Carbs: 12.68 g

103% FDI for Copper
94% FDI for Manganese
71% FDI for Fats - Polyunsaturated
63% FDI for Phosphorus
56% FDI for Iron
46% FDI for Riboflavin (Vitamin B2)
34% FDI for Protein
32% FDI for Magnesium
27% FDI for Vitamin B6
27% FDI for Niacin (Vitamin B3)
18% FDI for Calcium
17% FDI for Zinc
16% FDI for Fats - Saturated
15% FDI for Potassium
13% FDI for Fats - Monounsaturated
11% FDI for Thiamine (Vitamin B1)
10% FDI for Folate
9% FDI for Pantothenic Acid (Vitamin B5)
6% FDI for Carbohydrate
5% FDI for Vitamin B12

#7 Chickpea Flour (Besan)

Total Nutrient Score: 6.72
Overall Rank: 279 of 8990
Legumes Rank: 7 of 20
Serving Size: 1 cup (92 g)
Calories: 356 | Carbs: 53.19 g

101% FDI for Folate
93% FDI for Copper
64% FDI for Manganese
56% FDI for Iron
42% FDI for Phosphorus
37% FDI for Thiamine (Vitamin B1)
36% FDI for Magnesium
35% FDI for Vitamin B6
27% FDI for Fats - Polyunsaturated
26% FDI for Fiber
24% FDI for Carbohydrate
24% FDI for Zinc
21% FDI for Protein
17% FDI for Potassium
14% FDI for Selenium
11% FDI for Pantothenic Acid (Vitamin B5)
11% FDI for Vitamin K1
10% FDI for Niacin (Vitamin B3)
8% FDI for Riboflavin (Vitamin B2)
5% FDI for Vitamin E
4% FDI for Calcium
3% FDI for Fats - Monounsaturated
2% FDI for Fats - Saturated
1% FDI for Vitamin A

#8 Winged Beans

Total Nutrient Score: 6.12
Overall Rank: 364 of 8990
Legumes Rank: 8 of 20
Serving Size: 1 cup (172 g)
Cooking preparation: cooked, boiled, without salt
Calories: 253 | Carbs: 25.7 g

148% FDI for Copper
93% FDI for Iron
90% FDI for Manganese
42% FDI for Thiamine (Vitamin B1)
38% FDI for Phosphorus
27% FDI for Fats - Polyunsaturated
24% FDI for Calcium
23% FDI for Zinc
22% FDI for Magnesium
18% FDI for Protein
17% FDI for Riboflavin (Vitamin B2)
11% FDI for Carbohydrate
10% FDI for Potassium
9% FDI for Fats - Monounsaturated
9% FDI for Selenium
9% FDI for Niacin (Vitamin B3)
6% FDI for Vitamin B6
5% FDI for Pantothenic Acid (Vitamin B5)
5% FDI for Fats - Saturated
4% FDI for Folate

#9 Lentils

Total Nutrient Score: 5.96
Overall Rank: 388 of 8990
Legumes Rank: 9 of 20
Serving Size: 1 cup (198 g)
Cooking preparation: cooked, boiled, without salt
Calories: 230 | Carbs: 39.86 g

90% FDI for Folate
82% FDI for Iron
55% FDI for Copper
51% FDI for Phosphorus
43% FDI for Manganese
41% FDI for Fiber
28% FDI for Thiamine (Vitamin B1)
27% FDI for Vitamin B6
25% FDI for Pantothenic Acid (Vitamin B5)
23% FDI for Zinc
18% FDI for Protein
18% FDI for Carbohydrate
17% FDI for Magnesium
16% FDI for Potassium
13% FDI for Niacin (Vitamin B3)
12% FDI for Choline
11% FDI for Riboflavin (Vitamin B2)
10% FDI for Selenium
4% FDI for Vitamin K1
4% FDI for Calcium
3% FDI for Fats - Polyunsaturated
3% FDI for Vitamin C
1% FDI for Vitamin E

#10 Adzuki Beans

Total Nutrient Score: 5.87
Overall Rank: 405 of 8990
Legumes Rank: 10 of 20
Serving Size: 1 cup (230 g)
Cooking preparation: cooked, boiled, without salt
Calories: 294 | Carbs: 56.97 g

76% FDI for Copper
70% FDI for Folate
58% FDI for Iron
57% FDI for Manganese
55% FDI for Phosphorus
44% FDI for Fiber
37% FDI for Zinc
29% FDI for Magnesium
26% FDI for Potassium
25% FDI for Carbohydrate
22% FDI for Thiamine (Vitamin B1)
20% FDI for Pantothenic Acid (Vitamin B5)
17% FDI for Protein
17% FDI for Vitamin B6
11% FDI for Riboflavin (Vitamin B2)
10% FDI for Niacin (Vitamin B3)
6% FDI for Calcium
5% FDI for Selenium

#11 White Beans

Total Nutrient Score: 5.71
Overall Rank: 433 of 8990
Legumes Rank: 11 of 20
Serving Size: 1 cup (262 g)
Cooking preparation: canned
Calories: 299 | Carbs: 55.54 g

98% FDI for Iron
68% FDI for Copper
59% FDI for Manganese
43% FDI for Folate
34% FDI for Phosphorus
33% FDI for Fiber
32% FDI for Magnesium
27% FDI for Zinc
25% FDI for Potassium
25% FDI for Carbohydrate
21% FDI for Thiamine (Vitamin B1)
19% FDI for Calcium
19% FDI for Protein
15% FDI for Vitamin B6
14% FDI for Vitamin E
10% FDI for Pantothenic Acid (Vitamin B5)
10% FDI for Vitamin K1
8% FDI for Selenium
7% FDI for Riboflavin (Vitamin B2)
3% FDI for Fats - Polyunsaturated
2% FDI for Niacin (Vitamin B3)

#12 Navy Beans

Total Nutrient Score: 5.61
Overall Rank: 446 of 8990
Legumes Rank: 12 of 20
Serving Size: 1 cup (262 g)
Cooking preparation: canned
Calories: 296 | Carbs: 53.58 g

61% FDI for Iron
61% FDI for Copper
50% FDI for Phosphorus
43% FDI for Manganese
41% FDI for Folate
35% FDI for Fiber
31% FDI for Thiamine (Vitamin B1)
29% FDI for Magnesium
28% FDI for Selenium
24% FDI for Carbohydrate
21% FDI for Vitamin B6
20% FDI for Protein
18% FDI for Zinc
16% FDI for Potassium
14% FDI for Vitamin E
13% FDI for Choline
12% FDI for Calcium
11% FDI for Riboflavin (Vitamin B2)
10% FDI for Vitamin K1
9% FDI for Pantothenic Acid (Vitamin B5)
8% FDI for Niacin (Vitamin B3)
5% FDI for Fats - Polyunsaturated
2% FDI for Vitamin C
1% FDI for Fats - Saturated

#13 Great Northern Beans

Total Nutrient Score: 5.60
Overall Rank: 448 of 8990
Legumes Rank: 13 of 20
Serving Size: 1 cup (262 g)
Cooking preparation: canned
Calories: 299 | Carbs: 55.07 g

53% FDI for Folate
51% FDI for Iron
51% FDI for Phosphorus
47% FDI for Copper
46% FDI for Manganese
34% FDI for Fiber
32% FDI for Magnesium
31% FDI for Thiamine (Vitamin B1)
24% FDI for Carbohydrate
21% FDI for Vitamin B6
20% FDI for Potassium
19% FDI for Selenium
19% FDI for Protein
15% FDI for Zinc
15% FDI for Pantothenic Acid (Vitamin B5)
14% FDI for Choline
14% FDI for Calcium
14% FDI for Vitamin E
12% FDI for Riboflavin (Vitamin B2)
10% FDI for Vitamin K1
8% FDI for Niacin (Vitamin B3)
4% FDI for Fats - Polyunsaturated
4% FDI for Vitamin C
1% FDI for Fats - Saturated

#14 Chickpeas

Total Nutrient Score: 5.53
Overall Rank: 462 of 8990
Legumes Rank: 14 of 20
Serving Size: 1 cup (164 g)
Cooking preparation: cooked, boiled, without salt
Calories: 269 | Carbs: 44.97 g

73% FDI for Manganese
71% FDI for Folate
64% FDI for Copper
59% FDI for Iron
39% FDI for Phosphorus
33% FDI for Fiber
23% FDI for Zinc
20% FDI for Carbohydrate
19% FDI for Fats - Polyunsaturated
19% FDI for Magnesium
18% FDI for Vitamin B6
16% FDI for Thiamine (Vitamin B1)
15% FDI for Protein
13% FDI for Choline
11% FDI for Selenium
10% FDI for Potassium
9% FDI for Pantothenic Acid (Vitamin B5)
8% FDI for Vitamin K1
8% FDI for Calcium
8% FDI for Riboflavin (Vitamin B2)
5% FDI for Niacin (Vitamin B3)
4% FDI for Vitamin E
2% FDI for Fats - Monounsaturated
2% FDI for Vitamin C
2% FDI for Fats - Saturated
1% FDI for Vitamin A

#15 Baked Beans

Total Nutrient Score: 5.07
Overall Rank: 580 of 8990
Legumes Rank: 15 of 20
Serving Size: 1 cup (253 g)
Cooking preparation: home prepared
Calories: 392 | Carbs: 54.72 g

63% FDI for Iron
45% FDI for Copper
39% FDI for Phosphorus
37% FDI for Fiber
30% FDI for Folate
29% FDI for Thiamine (Vitamin B1)
28% FDI for Manganese
26% FDI for Selenium
26% FDI for Magnesium
24% FDI for Carbohydrate
19% FDI for Potassium
19% FDI for Fats - Polyunsaturated
18% FDI for Fats - Saturated
18% FDI for Vitamin B6
17% FDI for Zinc
15% FDI for Calcium
14% FDI for Protein
13% FDI for Fats - Monounsaturated
10% FDI for Riboflavin (Vitamin B2)
8% FDI for Pantothenic Acid (Vitamin B5)
6% FDI for Niacin (Vitamin B3)
3% FDI for Vitamin C

#16 Pink Beans

Total Nutrient Score: 5.01
Overall Rank: 607 of 8990
Legumes Rank: 16 of 20
Serving Size: 1 cup (169 g)
Cooking preparation: cooked, boiled, without salt
Calories: 252 | Carbs: 47.17 g

71% FDI for Folate
51% FDI for Copper
49% FDI for Iron
40% FDI for Manganese
40% FDI for Phosphorus
36% FDI for Thiamine (Vitamin B1)
26% FDI for Magnesium
24% FDI for Fiber
23% FDI for Vitamin B6
21% FDI for Carbohydrate
18% FDI for Potassium
15% FDI for Protein
15% FDI for Zinc
11% FDI for Choline
11% FDI for Vitamin E
10% FDI for Pantothenic Acid (Vitamin B5)
9% FDI for Calcium
8% FDI for Riboflavin (Vitamin B2)
8% FDI for Vitamin K1
6% FDI for Niacin (Vitamin B3)
4% FDI for Selenium
4% FDI for Fats - Polyunsaturated

#17 Pinto Beans

Total Nutrient Score: 4.97
Overall Rank: 626 of 8990
Legumes Rank: 17 of 20
Serving Size: 1 cup (171 g)
Cooking preparation: cooked, boiled, without salt
Calories: 245 | Carbs: 44.84 g

74% FDI for Folate
45% FDI for Iron
42% FDI for Copper
41% FDI for Fiber
36% FDI for Phosphorus
34% FDI for Manganese
30% FDI for Vitamin B6
28% FDI for Thiamine (Vitamin B1)
20% FDI for Magnesium
20% FDI for Carbohydrate
19% FDI for Selenium
16% FDI for Potassium
15% FDI for Protein
15% FDI for Zinc
11% FDI for Choline
11% FDI for Vitamin E
8% FDI for Riboflavin (Vitamin B2)
8% FDI for Calcium
8% FDI for Vitamin K1
7% FDI for Pantothenic Acid (Vitamin B5)
4% FDI for Fats - Polyunsaturated
3% FDI for Niacin (Vitamin B3)
2% FDI for Vitamin C

#18 Hyacinth Beans

Total Nutrient Score: 4.91
Overall Rank: 648 of 8990
Legumes Rank: 18 of 20
Serving Size: 1 cup (194 g)
Cooking preparation: cooked, boiled, without salt
Calories: 227 | Carbs: 40.14 g

111% FDI for Iron
74% FDI for Copper
50% FDI for Zinc
44% FDI for Thiamine (Vitamin B1)
41% FDI for Manganese
38% FDI for Magnesium
33% FDI for Phosphorus
18% FDI for Carbohydrate
16% FDI for Protein
14% FDI for Potassium
12% FDI for Pantothenic Acid (Vitamin B5)
10% FDI for Selenium
8% FDI for Calcium
6% FDI for Riboflavin (Vitamin B2)
6% FDI for Vitamin B6
5% FDI for Niacin (Vitamin B3)
5% FDI for Fats - Polyunsaturated
2% FDI for Folate

#19 Yellow Beans

Total Nutrient Score: 4.88
Overall Rank: 664 of 8990
Legumes Rank: 19 of 20
Serving Size: 1 cup (177 g)
Cooking preparation: cooked, boiled, without salt
Calories: 255 | Carbs: 44.75 g

55% FDI for Iron
48% FDI for Fiber
46% FDI for Phosphorus
37% FDI for Copper
36% FDI for Folate
35% FDI for Manganese
31% FDI for Magnesium
28% FDI for Thiamine (Vitamin B1)
20% FDI for Carbohydrate
18% FDI for Vitamin B6
17% FDI for Zinc
16% FDI for Protein
14% FDI for Riboflavin (Vitamin B2)
12% FDI for Potassium
11% FDI for Choline
11% FDI for Vitamin E
11% FDI for Calcium
8% FDI for Fats - Polyunsaturated
8% FDI for Pantothenic Acid (Vitamin B5)
8% FDI for Niacin (Vitamin B3)
8% FDI for Vitamin K1
4% FDI for Selenium
4% FDI for Vitamin C
2% FDI for Fats - Saturated

#20 Small White Beans

Total Nutrient Score: 4.84
Overall Rank: 683 of 8990
Legumes Rank: 20 of 20
Serving Size: 1 cup (179 g)
Cooking preparation: cooked, boiled, without salt
Calories: 254 | Carbs: 46.2 g

64% FDI for Iron
61% FDI for Folate
49% FDI for Fiber
43% FDI for Phosphorus
40% FDI for Manganese
35% FDI for Thiamine (Vitamin B1)
30% FDI for Copper
29% FDI for Magnesium
21% FDI for Carbohydrate
18% FDI for Zinc
18% FDI for Potassium
17% FDI for Vitamin B6
16% FDI for Protein
13% FDI for Calcium
9% FDI for Pantothenic Acid (Vitamin B5)
8% FDI for Riboflavin (Vitamin B2)
5% FDI for Fats - Polyunsaturated
4% FDI for Selenium
3% FDI for Niacin (Vitamin B3)
1% FDI for Fats - Saturated

GRAINS

Nutrients per One Serving

#1 Rice Bran

Total Nutrient Score: 28.91
Overall Rank: 9 of 8990
Grains Rank: 1 of 20
Serving Size: 1 cup (118 g)
Calories: 373 | Carbs: 58.63 g

729% FDI for Manganese *UL used for ranking analysis
369% FDI for Vitamin B6
283% FDI for Phosphorus
274% FDI for Iron
271% FDI for Thiamine (Vitamin B1)
251% FDI for Niacin (Vitamin B3)
220% FDI for Magnesium
174% FDI for Pantothenic Acid (Vitamin B5)
95% FDI for Copper
88% FDI for Fats - Polyunsaturated
65% FDI for Fiber
65% FDI for Zinc
39% FDI for Vitamin E
37% FDI for Potassium
33% FDI for Selenium
26% FDI for Carbohydrate
26% FDI for Riboflavin (Vitamin B2)
22% FDI for Fats - Monounsaturated
19% FDI for Folate
18% FDI for Fats - Saturated
16% FDI for Protein
7% FDI for Choline
7% FDI for Calcium
6% FDI for Lutein+Zeaxanthin
3% FDI for Vitamin K1

#2 Wheat Germ

Total Nutrient Score: 18.88
Overall Rank: 34 of 8990
Grains Rank: 2 of 20
Serving Size: 1 cup (115 g)
Calories: 414 | Carbs: 59.57 g

665% FDI for Manganese *UL used for ranking analysis
180% FDI for Thiamine (Vitamin B1)
166% FDI for Selenium
138% FDI for Phosphorus
128% FDI for Zinc
115% FDI for Vitamin B6
102% FDI for Copper
90% FDI for Iron
81% FDI for Folate
69% FDI for Fats - Polyunsaturated
65% FDI for Magnesium
52% FDI for Pantothenic Acid (Vitamin B5)
49% FDI for Niacin (Vitamin B3)
44% FDI for Riboflavin (Vitamin B2)
40% FDI for Fiber
27% FDI for Protein
26% FDI for Carbohydrate
22% FDI for Potassium
7% FDI for Fats - Saturated
5% FDI for Calcium
4% FDI for Fats - Monounsaturated

#3 Teff

Total Nutrient Score: 15.91
Overall Rank: 45 of 8990
Grains Rank: 3 of 20
Serving Size: 1 cup (193 g)
Calories: 708 | Carbs: 141.14 g

775% FDI for Manganese *UL used for ranking analysis
184% FDI for Iron
174% FDI for Copper
118% FDI for Phosphorus
85% FDI for Magnesium
72% FDI for Vitamin B6
64% FDI for Zinc
63% FDI for Thiamine (Vitamin B1)
63% FDI for Carbohydrate
41% FDI for Niacin (Vitamin B3)
41% FDI for Fiber
40% FDI for Riboflavin (Vitamin B2)
36% FDI for Pantothenic Acid (Vitamin B5)
35% FDI for Calcium
26% FDI for Protein
21% FDI for Fats - Polyunsaturated
18% FDI for Potassium
15% FDI for Selenium
5% FDI for Vitamin K1
5% FDI for Choline
3% FDI for Fats - Saturated
3% FDI for Lutein+Zeaxanthin
3% FDI for Fats - Monounsaturated
1% FDI for Vitamin E

#4 Amaranth Grain

Total Nutrient Score: 14.93
Overall Rank: 50 of 8990
Grains Rank: 4 of 20
Serving Size: 1 cup (193 g)
Calories: 716 | Carbs: 125.93 g

280% FDI for Manganese
184% FDI for Iron
154% FDI for Phosphorus
114% FDI for Magnesium
113% FDI for Copper
88% FDI for Vitamin B6
66% FDI for Selenium
56% FDI for Pantothenic Acid (Vitamin B5)
56% FDI for Carbohydrate
54% FDI for Fats - Polyunsaturated
50% FDI for Zinc
40% FDI for Folate
34% FDI for Fiber
31% FDI for Calcium
30% FDI for Riboflavin (Vitamin B2)
26% FDI for Protein
24% FDI for Choline
21% FDI for Potassium
19% FDI for Thiamine (Vitamin B1)
15% FDI for Vitamin E
11% FDI for Niacin (Vitamin B3)
10% FDI for Fats - Saturated
9% FDI for Vitamin C
8% FDI for Fats - Monounsaturated
1% FDI for Lutein+Zeaxanthin

#5 Wheat Durum

Total Nutrient Score: 14.63
Overall Rank: 52 of 8990
Grains Rank: 5 of 20
Serving Size: 1 cup (192 g)
Calories: 651 | Carbs: 136.57 g

312% FDI for Selenium
251% FDI for Manganese
139% FDI for Phosphorus
118% FDI for Copper
85% FDI for Iron
81% FDI for Niacin (Vitamin B3)
73% FDI for Zinc
67% FDI for Thiamine (Vitamin B1)
66% FDI for Magnesium
62% FDI for Vitamin B6
61% FDI for Carbohydrate
36% FDI for Pantothenic Acid (Vitamin B5)
26% FDI for Protein
21% FDI for Folate
19% FDI for Fats - Polyunsaturated
18% FDI for Riboflavin (Vitamin B2)
18% FDI for Potassium
7% FDI for Calcium
3% FDI for Fats - Saturated
2% FDI for Fats - Monounsaturated

#6 Wheat (Hard Red Spring, Hard Red Winter, or Hard White)

Total Nutrient Score: 14.52
Overall Rank: 53 of 8990
Grains Rank: 6 of 20
Serving Size: 1 cup (192 g)
Calories: 632 | Carbs: 130.62 g

339% FDI for Manganese
247% FDI for Selenium
91% FDI for Phosphorus
87% FDI for Copper 86% FDI for Iron
81% FDI for Thiamine (Vitamin B1)
69% FDI for Niacin (Vitamin B3)
62% FDI for Fiber
58% FDI for Carbohydrate
57% FDI for Magnesium
50% FDI for Vitamin B6
49% FDI for Zinc
36% FDI for Pantothenic Acid (Vitamin B5)
30% FDI for Protein
21% FDI for Folate
16% FDI for Riboflavin (Vitamin B2)
15% FDI for Fats - Polyunsaturated
14% FDI for Potassium
13% FDI for Vitamin E
11% FDI for Choline
10% FDI for Lutein+Zeaxanthin
5% FDI for Calcium
5% FDI for Vitamin K1
2% FDI for Fats - Saturated
1% FDI for Fats - Monounsaturated

#7 Quinoa

Total Nutrient Score: 11.94
Overall Rank: 81 of 8990
Grains Rank: 7 of 20
Serving Size: 1 cup (170 g)
Calories: 626 | Carbs: 109.07 g

150% FDI for Manganese
111% FDI for Copper
111% FDI for Phosphorus
97% FDI for Iron
80% FDI for Magnesium
78% FDI for Folate
64% FDI for Vitamin B6
56% FDI for Fats – Polyunsaturated
51% FDI for Thiamine (Vitamin B1)
48% FDI for Carbohydrate
48% FDI for Zinc
42% FDI for Riboflavin (Vitamin B2)
36% FDI for Omega-3 (DHA, 22:6)
31% FDI for Fiber
28% FDI for Vitamin E
26% FDI for Pantothenic Acid (Vitamin B5)
26% FDI for Selenium
24% FDI for Protein
22% FDI for Choline
20% FDI for Potassium
16% FDI for Niacin (Vitamin B3)
8% FDI for Calcium
7% FDI for Fats – Monounsaturated
7% FDI for Lutein+Zeaxanthin
4% FDI for Fats – Saturated

#8 Oats

Total Nutrient Score: 11.69
Overall Rank: 83 of 8990
Grains Rank: 8 of 20
Serving Size: 1 cup (156 g)
Calories: 607 | Carbs: 103.38 g

333% FDI for Manganese
117% FDI for Phosphorus
109% FDI for Copper
99% FDI for Thiamine (Vitamin B1)
92% FDI for Iron
66% FDI for Magnesium
56% FDI for Zinc
46% FDI for Carbohydrate
43% FDI for Fiber
42% FDI for Pantothenic Acid (Vitamin B5)
40% FDI for Fats – Polyunsaturated
26% FDI for Protein
22% FDI for Folate
17% FDI for Riboflavin (Vitamin B2)
14% FDI for Vitamin B6
14% FDI for Potassium
9% FDI for Niacin (Vitamin B3)
8% FDI for Fats – Monounsaturated
8% FDI for Calcium
7% FDI for Fats – Saturated

#9 Rye Flour

Total Nutrient Score: 11.47
Overall Rank: 88 of 8990
Grains Rank: 9 of 20
Serving Size: 1 cup (128 g)
Calories: 416 | Carbs: 87.85 g

337% FDI for Manganese
91% FDI for Phosphorus
80% FDI for Fiber
80% FDI for Copper
80% FDI for Iron
59% FDI for Zinc
49% FDI for Magnesium
44% FDI for Vitamin B6
42% FDI for Selenium
39% FDI for Carbohydrate
37% FDI for Pantothenic Acid (Vitamin B5)
34% FDI for Niacin (Vitamin B3)
34% FDI for Thiamine (Vitamin B1)
25% FDI for Riboflavin (Vitamin B2)
23% FDI for Vitamin E
20% FDI for Protein
20% FDI for Potassium
13% FDI for Fats - Polyunsaturated
11% FDI for Folate
10% FDI for Vitamin K1
7% FDI for Choline
6% FDI for Lutein+Zeaxanthin
5% FDI for Calcium
1% FDI for Fats - Saturated

#10 Granola

Total Nutrient Score: 11.36
Overall Rank: 91 of 8990
Grains Rank: 10 of 20
Serving Size: 1 cup (122 g)
Calories: 597 | Carbs: 65.73 g

212% FDI for Manganese
95% FDI for Fats - Polyunsaturated
90% FDI for Vitamin E
88% FDI for Copper
75% FDI for Phosphorus
60% FDI for Iron
56% FDI for Selenium
56% FDI for Thiamine (Vitamin B1)
49% FDI for Magnesium
46% FDI for Zinc
35% FDI for Vitamin B6
33% FDI for Fats - Monounsaturated
33% FDI for Riboflavin (Vitamin B2)
29% FDI for Carbohydrate
29% FDI for Fiber
26% FDI for Folate
21% FDI for Niacin (Vitamin B3)
18% FDI for Pantothenic Acid (Vitamin B5)
18% FDI for Fats - Saturated
17% FDI for Protein
14% FDI for Potassium
11% FDI for Choline
9% FDI for Calcium
8% FDI for Vitamin K1
4% FDI for Lutein+Zeaxanthin
2% FDI for Vitamin C

#11 Barley (hulled)

Total Nutrient Score: 11.33
Overall Rank: 92 of 8990
Grains Rank: 11 of 20
Serving Size: 1 cup (184 g)
Calories: 651 | Carbs: 135.2 g

155% FDI for Manganese
126% FDI for Selenium
102% FDI for Copper
99% FDI for Thiamine (Vitamin B1)
84% FDI for Fiber
83% FDI for Iron
69% FDI for Phosphorus
60% FDI for Carbohydrate
58% FDI for Magnesium
53% FDI for Niacin (Vitamin B3)
46% FDI for Zinc
45% FDI for Vitamin B6
40% FDI for Riboflavin (Vitamin B2)
23% FDI for Protein
20% FDI for Fats - Polyunsaturated
18% FDI for Potassium
10% FDI for Pantothenic Acid (Vitamin B5)
9% FDI for Folate
7% FDI for Vitamin E
7% FDI for Lutein+Zeaxanthin
6% FDI for Calcium
5% FDI for Vitamin K1
3% FDI for Fats - Saturated
1% FDI for Fats - Monounsaturated
1% FDI for Vitamin A

#12 Spelt

Total Nutrient Score: 10.95
Overall Rank: 99 of 8990
Grains Rank: 12 of 20
Serving Size: 1 cup (174 g)
Calories: 588 | Carbs: 122.13 g

226% FDI for Manganese
100% FDI for Phosphorus
99% FDI for Copper
97% FDI for Iron
74% FDI for Niacin (Vitamin B3)
56% FDI for Magnesium
54% FDI for Carbohydrate
53% FDI for Thiamine (Vitamin B1)
52% FDI for Zinc
49% FDI for Fiber
37% FDI for Pantothenic Acid (Vitamin B5)
37% FDI for Selenium
31% FDI for Vitamin B6
25% FDI for Protein
22% FDI for Fats - Polyunsaturated
20% FDI for Folate
15% FDI for Riboflavin (Vitamin B2)
14% FDI for Potassium
9% FDI for Vitamin E
8% FDI for Vitamin K1
7% FDI for Lutein+Zeaxanthin
5% FDI for Calcium
3% FDI for Fats - Saturated
2% FDI for Fats - Monounsaturated

#13 Millet

Total Nutrient Score: 10.65
Overall Rank: 104 of 8990
Grains Rank: 13 of 20
Serving Size: 1 cup (200 g)
Calories: 756 | Carbs: 145.7 g

167% FDI for Copper
142% FDI for Manganese
81% FDI for Phosphorus
75% FDI for Iron
70% FDI for Thiamine (Vitamin B1)
65% FDI for Carbohydrate
59% FDI for Vitamin B6
59% FDI for Niacin (Vitamin B3)
54% FDI for Magnesium
45% FDI for Fiber
45% FDI for Riboflavin (Vitamin B2)
43% FDI for Fats - Polyunsaturated
43% FDI for Folate
34% FDI for Pantothenic Acid (Vitamin B5)
31% FDI for Zinc
22% FDI for Protein
10% FDI for Selenium
8% FDI for Potassium
5% FDI for Fats - Saturated
4% FDI for Fats - Monounsaturated
2% FDI for Vitamin K1
2% FDI for Calcium

#14 Wheat (Soft Red Winter or Soft White)

Total Nutrient Score: 10.52
Overall Rank: 110 of 8990
Grains Rank: 14 of 20
Serving Size: 1 cup (168 g)
Calories: 556 | Carbs: 124.72 g

321% FDI for Manganese
118% FDI for Phosphorus
84% FDI for Copper
67% FDI for Iron
55% FDI for Carbohydrate
55% FDI for Fiber
55% FDI for Thiamine (Vitamin B1)
50% FDI for Magnesium
50% FDI for Niacin (Vitamin B3)
40% FDI for Zinc
35% FDI for Vitamin B6
29% FDI for Pantothenic Acid (Vitamin B5)
17% FDI for Protein
17% FDI for Folate
14% FDI for Potassium
12% FDI for Riboflavin (Vitamin B2)
11% FDI for Vitamin E
11% FDI for Fats - Polyunsaturated
5% FDI for Calcium
2% FDI for Fats - Saturated

#15 Triticale

Total Nutrient Score: 9.95
Overall Rank: 123 of 8990
Grains Rank: 15 of 20
Serving Size: 1 cup (192 g)
Calories: 645 | Carbs: 138.49 g

268% FDI for Manganese
98% FDI for Phosphorus
97% FDI for Copper
67% FDI for Thiamine (Vitamin B1)
62% FDI for Iron
62% FDI for Carbohydrate
60% FDI for Zinc
60% FDI for Magnesium
51% FDI for Pantothenic Acid (Vitamin B5)
35% FDI for Folate
25% FDI for Protein
20% FDI for Vitamin B6
20% FDI for Riboflavin (Vitamin B2)
18% FDI for Fats - Polyunsaturated
17% FDI for Niacin (Vitamin B3)
14% FDI for Potassium
12% FDI for Vitamin E
7% FDI for Calcium
3% FDI for Fats - Saturated
1% FDI for Fats - Monounsaturated

#16 Brown Rice (long grain)

Total Nutrient Score: 9.87
Overall Rank: 125 of 8990
Grains Rank: 16 of 20
Serving Size: 1 cup (185 g)
Calories: 679 | Carbs: 141.06 g

229% FDI for Manganese
83% FDI for Thiamine (Vitamin B1)
82% FDI for Phosphorus
75% FDI for Niacin (Vitamin B3)
68% FDI for Vitamin B6
63% FDI for Carbohydrate
62% FDI for Copper
57% FDI for Selenium
51% FDI for Magnesium
39% FDI for Pantothenic Acid (Vitamin B5)
36% FDI for Zinc
30% FDI for Iron
19% FDI for Fats - Polyunsaturated
18% FDI for Fiber
14% FDI for Protein
14% FDI for Riboflavin (Vitamin B2)
11% FDI for Folate
10% FDI for Potassium
7% FDI for Vitamin E
7% FDI for Choline
5% FDI for Fats - Monounsaturated
4% FDI for Fats - Saturated
2% FDI for Calcium
1% FDI for Vitamin K1

#17 Buckwheat

Total Nutrient Score: 9.86
Overall Rank: 127 of 8990
Grains Rank: 17 of 20
Serving Size: 1 cup (170 g)
Calories: 583 | Carbs: 121.55 g

208% FDI for Copper
96% FDI for Manganese
94% FDI for Magnesium
84% FDI for Phosphorus
75% FDI for Niacin (Vitamin B3)
56% FDI for Riboflavin (Vitamin B2)
54% FDI for Carbohydrate
47% FDI for Iron
45% FDI for Fiber
42% FDI for Pantothenic Acid (Vitamin B5)
37% FDI for Zinc
27% FDI for Vitamin B6
26% FDI for Selenium
23% FDI for Protein
18% FDI for Fats - Polyunsaturated
17% FDI for Potassium
14% FDI for Thiamine (Vitamin B1)
13% FDI for Folate
5% FDI for Fats - Saturated
4% FDI for Fats - Monounsaturated
3% FDI for Calcium

#18 Rye Grain

Total Nutrient Score: 9.67
Overall Rank: 130 of 8990
Grains Rank: 18 of 20
Serving Size: 1 cup (169 g)
Calories: 571 | Carbs: 128.2 g

189% FDI for Manganese
80% FDI for Phosphorus
69% FDI for Copper
67% FDI for Fiber
57% FDI for Carbohydrate
56% FDI for Iron
49% FDI for Pantothenic Acid (Vitamin B5)
45% FDI for Niacin (Vitamin B3)
45% FDI for Thiamine (Vitamin B1)
44% FDI for Magnesium
43% FDI for Selenium
41% FDI for Zinc
38% FDI for Vitamin B6
33% FDI for Riboflavin (Vitamin B2)
18% FDI for Potassium
17% FDI for Protein
16% FDI for Folate
13% FDI for Fats - Polyunsaturated
13% FDI for Vitamin K1
10% FDI for Vitamin E
9% FDI for Choline
8% FDI for Lutein+Zeaxanthin
4% FDI for Calcium
1% FDI for Fats - Saturated

#19 Oat Bran

Total Nutrient Score: 9.11
Overall Rank: 140 of 8990
Grains Rank: 19 of 20
Serving Size: 1 cup (94 g)
Calories: 231 | Carbs: 62.25 g

230% FDI for Manganese
99% FDI for Phosphorus
92% FDI for Thiamine (Vitamin B1)
77% FDI for Selenium
64% FDI for Iron
53% FDI for Magnesium
42% FDI for Copper
38% FDI for Fiber
28% FDI for Pantothenic Acid (Vitamin B5)
28% FDI for Carbohydrate
27% FDI for Zinc
26% FDI for Fats - Polyunsaturated
16% FDI for Protein
16% FDI for Riboflavin (Vitamin B2)
12% FDI for Folate
12% FDI for Vitamin B6
11% FDI for Potassium
6% FDI for Vitamin E
6% FDI for Fats - Monounsaturated
6% FDI for Choline
6% FDI for Calcium
5% FDI for Niacin (Vitamin B3)
5% FDI for Fats - Saturated
4% FDI for Lutein+Zeaxanthin
4% FDI for Vitamin K1

#20 Brown Rice Flour

Total Nutrient Score: 9.10
Overall Rank: 141 of 8990
Grains Rank: 20 of 20
Serving Size: 1 cup (158 g)
Calories: 574 | Carbs: 120.84 g

276% FDI for Manganese
89% FDI for Vitamin B6
76% FDI for Phosphorus
63% FDI for Niacin (Vitamin B3)
58% FDI for Thiamine (Vitamin B1)
54% FDI for Carbohydrate
50% FDI for Pantothenic Acid (Vitamin B5)
42% FDI for Magnesium
40% FDI for Copper
39% FDI for Iron
35% FDI for Zinc
19% FDI for Fiber
16% FDI for Fats - Polyunsaturated
11% FDI for Protein
10% FDI for Potassium
10% FDI for Riboflavin (Vitamin B2)
6% FDI for Vitamin E
6% FDI for Folate
4% FDI for Fats - Monounsaturated
3% FDI for Fats - Saturated
2% FDI for Calcium

FATS AND OILS

Nutrients per One Serving

#1 Salmon Oil

Total Nutrient Score: 20.07
Overall Rank: 26 of 8990
Fats and Oils Rank: 1 of 20
Serving Size: 1 tbsp (13.6 g)
Calories: 123 | Carbs: 0 g

1127% FDI for Omega-3 (DHA, 22:6)
805% FDI for Omega-3 (EPA, 20:5)
55% FDI for Fats - Polyunsaturated
10% FDI for Fats - Saturated
10% FDI for Fats - Monounsaturated

#2 Menhaden Oil

Total Nutrient Score: 14.14
Overall Rank: 57 of 8990
Fats and Oils Rank: 2 of 20
Serving Size: 1 tbsp (13.6 g)
Calories: 123 | Carbs: 0 g

814% FDI for Omega-3 (EPA, 20:5)
529% FDI for Omega-3 (DHA, 22:6)
47% FDI for Fats - Polyunsaturated
15% FDI for Fats - Saturated
9% FDI for Fats - Monounsaturated

#3 Sardine Oil

Total Nutrient Score: 13.55
Overall Rank: 66 of 8990
Fats and Oils Rank: 3 of 20
Serving Size: 1 tbsp (13.6 g)
Calories: 123 | Carbs: 0 g

659% FDI for Omega-3 (DHA, 22:6)
627% FDI for Omega-3 (EPA, 20:5)
43% FDI for Fats - Polyunsaturated
15% FDI for Fats - Saturated
12% FDI for Fats - Monounsaturated

#4 Herring Oil

Total Nutrient Score: 6.99
Overall Rank: 261 of 8990
Fats and Oils Rank: 4 of 20
Serving Size: 1 tbsp (13.6 g)
Calories: 123 | Carbs: 0 g

388% FDI for Omega-3 (EPA, 20:5)
260% FDI for Omega-3 (DHA, 22:6)
21% FDI for Fats - Polyunsaturated
19% FDI for Fats - Monounsaturated
11% FDI for Fats - Saturated

#5 Cod Liver Oil

Total Nutrient Score: 5.35
Overall Rank: 504 of 8990
Fats and Oils Rank: 5 of 20
Serving Size: 1 tsp (4.5 g)
Calories: 41 | Carbs: 0 g

225% FDI for Omega-3 (DHA, 22:6)
150% FDI for Vitamin A
141% FDI for Omega-3 (EPA, 20:5)
10% FDI for Fats - Polyunsaturated
5% FDI for Fats - Monounsaturated
4% FDI for Fats - Saturated

#6 Safflower Oil (linoleic, over 70%)

Total Nutrient Score: 1.42
Overall Rank: 3575 of 8990
Fats and Oils Rank: 6 of 20
Serving Size: 1 tbsp (13.6 g)
Calories: 120 | Carbs: 0 g

101% FDI for Fats - Polyunsaturated
31% FDI for Vitamin E
5% FDI for Fats - Monounsaturated
3% FDI for Fats - Saturated
1% FDI for Vitamin K1

#7 Grapeseed Oil

Total Nutrient Score: 1.32
Overall Rank: 3683 of 8990
Fats and Oils Rank: 7 of 20
Serving Size: 1 tablespoon (13.6 g)
Calories: 120 | Carbs: 0 g

95% FDI for Fats - Polyunsaturated
26% FDI for Vitamin E
5% FDI for Fats - Monounsaturated
5% FDI for Fats - Saturated

#8 Cottonseed Oil

Total Nutrient Score: 1.26
Overall Rank: 3734 of 8990
Fats and Oils Rank: 8 of 20
Serving Size: 1 tablespoon (13.6 g)
Calories: 120 | Carbs: 0 g

71% FDI for Fats - Polyunsaturated
32% FDI for Vitamin E
13% FDI for Fats - Saturated
6% FDI for Fats - Monounsaturated
4% FDI for Vitamin K1

#9 Poppyseed Oil

Total Nutrient Score: 1.09
Overall Rank: 4053 of 8990
Fats and Oils Rank: 9 of 20
Serving Size: 1 tablespoon (13.6 g)
Calories: 120 | Carbs: 0 g

85% FDI for Fats - Polyunsaturated
10% FDI for Vitamin E
7% FDI for Fats - Saturated
7% FDI for Fats - Monounsaturated

#10 Flaxseed Oil (cold pressed)

Total Nutrient Score: 1.05
Overall Rank: 4143 of 8990
Fats and Oils Rank: 10 of 20
Serving Size: 1 tbsp (13.6 g)
Calories: 120 | Carbs: 0 g

92% FDI for Fats - Polyunsaturated
6% FDI for Fats - Monounsaturated
5% FDI for Fats - Saturated
2% FDI for Vitamin K1

#11 Rice Bran Oil

Total Nutrient Score: 1.05
Overall Rank: 4152 of 8990
Fats and Oils Rank: 11 of 20
Serving Size: 1 tablespoon (13.6 g)
Calories: 120 | Carbs: 0 g

48% FDI for Fats - Polyunsaturated
29% FDI for Vitamin E
13% FDI for Fats - Monounsaturated
10% FDI for Fats - Saturated
4% FDI for Vitamin K1

#12 Walnut Oil

Total Nutrient Score: 1.01
Overall Rank: 4204 of 8990
Fats and Oils Rank: 12 of 20
Serving Size: 1 tbsp (13.6 g)
Calories: 120 | Carbs: 0 g

86% FDI for Fats - Polyunsaturated
8% FDI for Fats - Monounsaturated
5% FDI for Fats - Saturated
3% FDI for Vitamin K1

#13 Oat Oil

Total Nutrient Score: 0.95
Overall Rank: 4330 of 8990
Fats and Oils Rank: 13 of 20
Serving Size: 1 tbsp (13.6 g)
Calories: 120 | Carbs: 0 g

56% FDI for Fats - Polyunsaturated
13% FDI for Vitamin E
12% FDI for Fats - Monounsaturated
10% FDI for Fats - Saturated
4% FDI for Vitamin K1

#14 Canola Oil

Total Nutrient Score: 0.94
Overall Rank: 4344 of 8990
Fats and Oils Rank: 14 of 20
Serving Size: 1 tbsp (14 g)
Calories: 124 | Carbs: 0 g

39% FDI for Fats - Polyunsaturated
22% FDI for Fats - Monounsaturated
16% FDI for Vitamin E
13% FDI for Vitamin K1
4% FDI for Fats - Saturated

#15 Tomatoseed Oil

Total Nutrient Score: 0.93
Overall Rank: 4355 of 8990
Fats and Oils Rank: 15 of 20
Serving Size: 1 tablespoon (13.6 g)
Calories: 120 | Carbs: 0 g

72% FDI for Fats - Polyunsaturated
10% FDI for Fats - Saturated
8% FDI for Fats - Monounsaturated
3% FDI for Vitamin E

#16 Almond Oil

Total Nutrient Score: 0.88
Overall Rank: 4439 of 8990
Fats and Oils Rank: 16 of 20
Serving Size: 1 tablespoon (13.6 g)
Calories: 120 | Carbs: 0 g

36% FDI for Vitamin E
24% FDI for Fats - Monounsaturated
24% FDI for Fats - Polyunsaturated
4% FDI for Fats - Saturated
1% FDI for Vitamin K1

#17 Hazelnut Oil

Total Nutrient Score: 0.87
Overall Rank: 4467 of 8990
Fats and Oils Rank: 17 of 20
Serving Size: 1 tablespoon (13.6 g)
Calories: 120 | Carbs: 0 g

43% FDI for Vitamin E
27% FDI for Fats - Monounsaturated
14% FDI for Fats - Polyunsaturated
4% FDI for Fats - Saturated

#18 Peanut Oil

Total Nutrient Score: 0.82
Overall Rank: 4553 of 8990
Fats and Oils Rank: 18 of 20
Serving Size: 1 tbsp (13.5 g)
Calories: 119 | Carbs: 0 g

43% FDI for Fats - Polyunsaturated
16% FDI for Fats - Monounsaturated
14% FDI for Vitamin E
8% FDI for Fats - Saturated

#19 Sesame Oil

Total Nutrient Score: 0.81
Overall Rank: 4562 of 8990
Fats and Oils Rank: 19 of 20
Serving Size: 1 tablespoon (13.6 g)
Calories: 120 | Carbs: 0 g

57% FDI for Fats - Polyunsaturated
13% FDI for Fats - Monounsaturated
7% FDI for Fats - Saturated
2% FDI for Vitamin K1
1% FDI for Vitamin E

#20 Wheat Germ Oil

Total Nutrient Score: 0.79
Overall Rank: 4588 of 8990
Fats and Oils Rank: 20 of 20
Serving Size: 1 tsp (4.5 g)
Calories: 40 | Carbs: 0 g

45% FDI for Vitamin E
28% FDI for Fats - Polyunsaturated
3% FDI for Fats - Saturated
2% FDI for Fats - Monounsaturated
1% FDI for Vitamin K1

REFERENCES

1. "FDA Cuts Trans Fat In Processed Foods." U.S. Food & Drug Administration. 15 June 2015. Web. 26 Dec 2016. http://www.fda.gov/ForConsumers/ConsumerUpdates/ucm372915.htm.

2. Butler, Natalie. "Nutritional Deficiencies (Malnutrition)." Healthline. 6 Nov. 2015. Web. 13 Dec 2016. http://www.healthline.com/health/malnutrition#Treatment6.

3. Geleijnse, Johanna M. et al. "Dietary Intake of Menaquinone is Associated with a Reduced Risk of Coronary Heart Disease: The Rotterdam Study." The Journal of Nutrition 134.11 (2004): 3100-3105. http://jn.nutrition.org/content/134/11/3100.full.

4. Nakamura, Eriko et al. "Low-Dose Menaquinone-4 Improves γ-Carboxylation of Osteocalcin in Young Males: A Non-Placebo-Controlled Dose–response Study." Nutrition Journal 13 (2014): 85. PMC. Web. 16 Dec 2016. https://www.ncbi.nlm.nih.gov/pubmed/25163392.

5. Scientific Panel on Dietetic Products, Nutrition and Allergies. "Tolerable Upper Intake Levels for Vitamins and Minerals." European Food and Safety Authority. Scientific Committee on Food, Feb. 2006. Web. 14 Sept. 2015. http://www.efsa.europa.eu/sites/default/files/efsa_rep/blobserver_assets/ndatolerableuil.pdf.

6. Suttie, J.W. Fat Soluble Vitamins: Their Biochemistry & Applications. Boca Raton: CRC Press, 1985. 225-311.

7. Geleijnse, Johanna M. et. al. "Dietary Intake of Menaquinone Is Associated with a Reduced Risk of Coronary Heart Disease: The Rotterdam Study." Journal of Nutrition 134.11 (2004): 3100-3105. Web. 16 Dec 2016. https://www.ncbi.nlm.nih.gov/pubmed/15514282.

8. Cockayne, S., Adamson, J., Lanham-New, S., Shearer, M.J., Gilbody, S. Torgerson, DJ. "Vitamin K and the prevention of fractures: systematic review and meta-analysis of randomized controlled trials." US National Library of Medicine National Institutes of Health. https://www.ncbi.nlm.nih.gov/pubmed/16801507.

9. Sato, Toshiro, Leon J Schurgers, and Kazuhiro Uenishi. "Comparison of Menaquinone-4 and Menaquinone-7 Bioavailability in Healthy Women." Nutrition Journal 11 (2012): 93. PMC. Web. 6 Jan 2016. http://www.ncbi.nlm.nih.gov/pubmed/23140417.

10. Mercola, Dr. Joseph & Droege, Rachael. "Fight Cancer With Vitamin K." 8 Oct. 2003. Web. 10 Nov 2016. http://articles.mercola.com/sites/articles/archive/2003/10/08/cancer-vitamin-k.aspx.

11. Asprey, Dave. "Upgrade Your Energy, Optimize Your Supplements." Bulletproof. 12 June 2012. Web. 6 Nov 2015. https://blog.bulletproof.com/optimize-your-supplements/.

12. Masterjohn, Chris. "The Daily Lipid Podcast Episode 18: You Asked Me Anything About Fat-Soluble Vitamins, Facebook Live, 06/29/16." Chris Masterjohn, PhD. 2 July 2016. Web. 19 Dec 2016. https://chrismasterjohnphd.com/2016/07/02/the-daily-lipid-podcast-episode-18-you-asked-me-anything-about-fat-soluble-vitamins-facebook-live-062916/.

13. Kutty, Vin. "How to choose the right Vitamin K2 supplement." Omega Via. 23 April 2015. Web. 19 Dec 2016. http://omegavia.com/how-to-choose-the-right-vitamin-k2-supplement/.

14. Zeisel, Steven H., da Costa, KA. "Choline: an essential nutrient for public health." US National Library of Medicine National Institutes of Health. http://www.ncbi.nlm.nih.gov/pubmed/19906248.

15. Institute of Medicine (US) Committee to Review Dietary Reference Intakes for Vitamin D and Calcium. "Dietary Reference Intakes (DRIs): Recommended Dietary Allowances and Adequate Intakes, Vitamins." Dietary Reference Intakes for Calcium and Vitamin D. Ed. Catherine A. Ross, Christine L. Taylor, Ann L. Yaktine, et al. National Academies Press, 2011. https://www.ncbi.nlm.nih.gov/books/NBK56068/table/summarytables.t2/.

16. Institute of Medicine (US) Committee to Review Dietary Reference Intakes for Vitamin D and Calcium. "Dietary Reference Intakes (DRIs): Tolerable Upper Intake Levels, Vitamins." Dietary Reference Intakes for Calcium and Vitamin D. Ed. Catherine A. Ross, Christine L. Taylor, Ann L. Yaktine, et al. National Academies Press, 2011. https://www.ncbi.nlm.nih.gov/books/NBK56068/table/summarytables.t7.

17. Food and Nutrition Board, Institute of Medicine. "DRI Dietary Reference Intakes for Thiamin, Riboflavin, Niacin, Vitamin B6, Folate, Vitamin B12, Pantothenic Acid, Biotin, and Choline." Washington, DC: National Academy Press, 2005. 115, 273, 281. https://www.nap.edu/read/6015/chapter/1.

18. U.S. Department of Health & Human Services. "Folate: Dietary Supplement Fact Sheet." National Institutes of Health. 20 April 2016. Web. 1 Jan 2017. https://ods.od.nih.gov/factsheets/Folate-HealthProfessional/.

19. Institute of Medicine (US) Committee to Review Dietary Reference Intakes for Vitamin D and Calcium. "Dietary Reference Intakes (DRIs): Recommended Dietary Allowances and Adequate Intakes, Elements." Dietary Reference Intakes for Calcium and Vitamin D. Ed. Catherine A. Ross, Christine L. Taylor, Ann L. Yaktine, et al. National Academies Press, 2011. https://www.ncbi.nlm.nih.gov/books/NBK56068/table/summarytables.t3.

20. Institute of Medicine (US) Committee to Review Dietary Reference Intakes for Vitamin D and Calcium. "Dietary Reference Intakes (DRIs): Tolerable Upper Intake Levels, Elements." Dietary Reference Intakes for Calcium and Vitamin D. Ed. Catherine A. Ross, Christine L. Taylor, Ann L. Yaktine, et al. National Academies Press, 2011. https://www.ncbi.nlm.nih.gov/books/NBK56068/table/summarytables.t8.

21. Kresser, Chris. "Episode 2 – essential fatty acids, fish & fish oil." Chris Kresser. 27 May 2010. Web. 18 Nov 2016. https://chriskresser.com/podcast-episode-ii-essential-fatty-acids-fish-and-fish-oil/.

22. "DHA/EPA and the Omega-3 Nutrition Gap/ Recommended Intakes." DHA-EPA Omega-3 Institute. Web. 16 Dec 2016. http://www.dhaomega3.org/Overview/DHAEPA-and-the-Omega-3-Nutrition-Gap-Recommended-Intakes.

23. Simopoulos, Artemis P. et. al. "Workshop on the essentiality of and recommended dietary intakes for omega-6 and omega-3 Fatty acids." Asia Pacific J Clin Nutr 8.4 (1999): 300-301. Web. 16 Dec 2016. https://www.ncbi.nlm.nih.gov/pubmed/24394233.

24. Gebauer, Sarah K. et. al. "n–3 Fatty acid dietary recommendations and food sources to achieve essentiality and cardiovascular benefits." American Journal of Clinical Nutrition 83.6 (2006): S1526-1535S.Web. 15 Dec 2016. http://ajcn.nutrition.org/content/83/6/S1526.long.

25. "Omega-3 fatty acids, fish oil, alpha-linolenic acid." Mayo Clinic. Web. 15 Dec 2016. http://www.mayoclinic.org/drugs-supplements/omega-3-fatty-acids-fish-oil-alpha-linolenic-acid/dosing/hrb-20059372.

26. Kresser, Chris. "When it comes to fish oil, more is not better." Chris Kresser. 25 Oct. 2010. Web. 19 Nov 2016. https://chriskresser.com/when-it-comes-to-fish-oil-more-is-not-better/.

27. Venturini, D.; Simão, A.N.; Urbano, M.R.; Dichi, I. Effects of extra virgin olive oil and fish oil on lipid profile and oxidative stress in patients with metabolic syndrome. Nutrition 2015, 31, 834–840. http://www.ncbi.nlm.nih.gov/pubmed/25933490.

28. Weil, Dr. Andrew. "Too Much Omega-3?" Dr. Weil. 27 Jan. 2012. Web. 18 Nov 2016. http://www.drweil.com/vitamins-supplements-herbs/vitamins/too-much-omega-3/.

29. "Fats: Total Fat & Fatty Acids." Australian Government National Health and Medical Research Council. 4 Sept. 2014. Web. 15 Dec 2016. https://www.nrv.gov.au/nutrients/fats-total-fat-fatty-acids.

30. Kresser, Chris. "9 Steps to Perfect Health - #4: Supplement Wisely." Chris Kresser. 18 Feb. 2011. Web. 6 Nov 2015. https://chriskresser.com/9-steps-to-perfect-health-4-supplement-wisely/

31. "How do I get the vitamin D my body needs?" Vitamin D Council. Web. 20 Nov. 2016. http://www.vitamindcouncil.org/about-vitamin-d/how-to-get-your-vitamin-d/vitamin-d-supplementation/.

32. "Pancreatic Cancer." Vitamin D Council. Web. 13 Dec. 2016. https://www.vitamindcouncil.org/health-conditions/pancreatic-cancer/.

33. Cannell, John. "What is the Upper Limit and NOAEL and are they Justified?" Vitamin D Council. Web. 5 Nov 2016 https://www.vitamindcouncil.org/what-is-the-upper-limit-and-noael-and-are-they-justified/.

34. DeLuca, Hector F., Prahl, Jean M., & Plum, Lori A. "1,25-Dihydroxyvitamin D is not responsible for toxicity caused by vitamin D or 25-hydroxyvitamin D." Archives of Biochemistry and Biophysics 505.2 (2011): 226-230. Web. 13 Dec 2016. https://www.ncbi.nlm.nih.gov/pubmed/20965147.

35. Kresser, Chris. "Vitamin D: More Is Not Better." Chris Kresser. 2 Aug. 2016. Web. 13 Dec 2016. https://chriskresser.com/vitamin-d-more-is-not-better/.

36. Institute of Medicine Committee to Review Dietary Reference Intakes for Vitamin D and Calcium. Dietary Reference Intakes for Calcium and Vitamin D. Washington, DC: National Academies Press, 2011. Web. 20 Dec 2016. https://www.ncbi.nlm.nih.gov/books/NBK56058/.

37. "How do I get the Vitamin D my Body Needs?" Vitamin D Council. Web. 8 Jan 2017. https://www.vitamindcouncil.org/about-vitamin-d/how-do-i-get-the-vitamin-d-my-body-needs/.

38. "Am I Getting Too Much Vitamin D?" Vitamin D Council. Web. 8 Jan 2017. https://www.vitamindcouncil.org/about-vitamin-d/am-i-getting-too-much-vitamin-d/.

39. GRACE Communications Foundation. "Soil Quality." www.sustainabletable.org. Web. 13 Dec 2016. http://www.sustainabletable.org/207/soil-quality.

40. U.S. Department of Health & Human Services. "Magnesium: Fact Sheet for Health Professionals." National Institutes of Health. 11 Feb. 2016. Web. 13 Dec 2016. https://ods.od.nih.gov/factsheets/Magnesium-HealthProfessional/#h8.

41. Institute of Medicine (US) Committee to Review Dietary Reference Intakes for Vitamin D and Calcium. "Dietary Reference Intakes (DRIs): Recommended Dietary Allowances and Adequate Intakes, Total Water and Macronutrients." Dietary Reference Intakes for Calcium and Vitamin D. Ed. Catherine A. Ross, Christine L. Taylor, Ann L. Yaktine, et al. National Academies Press, 2011. ttps://www.ncbi.nlm.nih.gov/books/NBK56068/table/summarytables.t4.

42. Turner, Nancy D. & Lupton, Joanne R. "Dietary Fiber." Advances in Nutrition 2. (2011): 151-152. Web. 14 Dec 2016. http://advances.nutrition.org/content/2/2/151.full.

43. Myhre, Anne M. et al. "Water-miscible, emulsified, and solid forms of retinol supplements are more toxic than oil-based preparations." American Journal of Clinical Nutrition 78.6 (2003): 1152-1159. Web. 5 Jan 2016. http://ajcn.nutrition.org/content/78/6/1152.long.

44. Masterjohn, Christopher. "Vitamin A On Trial: Does Vitamin A Cause Osteoporosis?" The Weston A. Price Foundation. 2 Aug 2006. Web. 20 Jan 2016. http://www.westonaprice.org/health-topics/abcs-of-nutrition/vitamin-a-on-trial-does-vitamin-a-cause-osteoporosis/.

45. Kresser, Chris. "5 Primal Superfoods for Fertility and Pregnancy." Chris Kresser. 2 May 2012. Web. 13 Dec 2016. http://www.marksdailyapple.com/5-primal-superfoods-for-fertility-and-pregnancy/.

46. Food and Nutrition Board Institute of Medicine. "Dietary Reference Intakes (DRIs): Tolerable. Upper Intake Levels, Vitamins." National Academies. Web. 6 June 2015. https://www.nationalacademies.org/hmd/~/media/Files/Activity%20Files/Nutrition/DRI-Tables/4_%20UL%20Values_Vitamins%20and%20Elements.pdf?la=en.

47. Zelman, Kathleen M. "Know the Difference Between Fat- and Water-Soluble Nutrients." WebMD. Web. 2 June 2015. http://www.webmd.com/vitamins-and-supplements/nutrition-vitamins-11/fat-water-nutrient.

48. Institute of Medicine (US) Panel on Dietary Antioxidants and Related Compounds. "Dietary Reference Intakes for Vitamin C, Vitamin E, Selenium, and Carotenoids." National Academies Press, 2000. https://www.ncbi.nlm.nih.gov/books/NBK225483/.

49. Chen F, Hu J, Liu P, Li J, Wei Z, Liu P. "Carotenoid intake and risk of non-Hodgkin lymphoma: a systematic review and dose-response meta-analysis of observational studies." US National Library of Medicine National Institutes of Health. 24 Dec 2016. Web. 2 Jan 2017. https://www.ncbi.nlm.nih.gov/pubmed/28011986.

50. Institute of Medicine. Dietary Reference Intakes for Vitamin C, Vitamin E, Selenium, and Carotenoids. Washington: DC, 2010. 246-247. https://www.nap.edu/read/9810/chapter/10#366.

51. Mannisto, Satu et. al. "Dietary Carotenoids and Risk of Lung Cancer in a Pooled Analysis of Seven Cohort Studies." American Association for Cancer Research 13.1 (2004): 40-48. Web. 11 Jan 2017. http://cebp.aacrjournals.org/content/13/1/40.full.

52. Li, Chaoyang et. al. "Serum α-carotene Concentrations and Risk of Death Among US Adults: The Third National Health and Nutrition Examination Survey Follow-up Study. Arch Intern Med 171.6 (2011): 507-15. Web. 12 Jan 2017. https://www.ncbi.nlm.nih.gov/pubmed/21098341.

53. Liu, Chun et al. "β-Cryptoxanthin Supplementation Prevents Cigarette Smoke-Induced Lung Inflammation, Oxidative Damage and Squamous Metaplasia in Ferrets." Cancer Prevention Research 4.8 (2011): 1255–1266. Web. 15 Dec 2016. https://www.ncbi.nlm.nih.gov/pmc/articles/PMC3151338/.

54. Chun Liu, Roderick T. Bronson, Robert M. Russell and Xiang-Dong Wang. "Beta-Cryptoxanthin Supplementation Prevents Cigarette Smoke-Induced Lung Inflammation, Oxidative Damage, and Squamous Metaplasia in Ferrets." Cancer Prev Res August 1 2011 (4) (8) 1255-1266; DOI: 10.1158/1940-6207.CAPR-10-0384 http://cancerpreventionresearch.aacrjournals.org/content/4/8/1255.full.

55. Yuan JM, Stram DO, Arakawa K, Lee HP, Yu MC. "Dietary cryptoxanthin and reduced risk of lung cancer: The Singapore Chinese Health Study." US National Library of Medicine National Institutes of Health. 12 Sept 2003. Web. 1 Jan 2017. https://www.ncbi.nlm.nih.gov/pubmed/14504200.

56. Devaraj, Sridevi et al. "A Dose-Response Study on the Effects of Purified Lycopene Supplementation on Biomarkers of Oxidative Stress." Journal of the American College ofNutrition 27.2 (2008): 267–273. http://www.ncbi.nlm.nih.gov/pmc/articles/PMC2677959.

57. Shao, Andrew & Hathcock, John N. "Risk Assessment for the Carotenoids Lutein and Lycopene." Regulatory Toxicology and Pharmacology 45.3 (2006): 289-298. Web. 12 Jan 2017. https://www.ncbi.nlm.nih.gov/pubmed/16814439.

58. Rosa, Alvarez-Parrilla, Gonzalez-Aguilar. Fruit and Vegetable Phytochemicals: Chemistry, Nutritional Value and Stability. Ames: Blackwell Publishing. 2010. 246-247.

59. Rao, A.V. & Honglei, Shen. "Effect of Low Dose Lycopene Intake on Lycopene Bioavailability and Oxidative Stress." Nutrition Research 22.10 (2002): 1125-1131. Web. 15 Dec 2016. http://www.nrjournal.com/article/S0271-5317(02)00430-X/abstract.

60. Welter, Melissa L. "The Effects of Lycopene on Your Health." North Dakota State University. Web. 1 Jan 2017. https://www.ndsu.edu/pubweb/chiwonlee/plsc211/student%20papers/articles04/Melissa%20Welter/mwelter.htm.

61. US Department of Health & Human Services. "Chapter 6 Overview." Dietary Guidelines for Americans 2005." 9 July 2008. Web. 22 Dec 2016. 19 Dec 2016. https://health.gov/dietaryguidelines/dga2005/document/html/chapter6.htm.

62. Food and Nutrition Board, Institute of Medicine. "Dietary reference intakes for Energy, Carbohydrate, Fiber, Fat, Fatty Acids, Cholesterol, Protein, and Amino Acids." Washington, DC: National Academy Press, 2005. 265, 422, 589, 645. https://www.nap.edu/read/10490/chapter/1#ii.

63. Mercola, Dr. Joseph. "To Achieve Optimal Health, Eat 50-70% of This Frequently Demonized Food." Mercola. 28 Dec. 2011. Web. 23 Dec 2016. http://articles.mercola.com/sites/articles/archive/2011/12/28/what-you-dont-know-about-fats.aspx.

64. Jaminet, Paul. "Hunter-Gatherer Macronutrient Ratios: More Data." Perfect Health Diet. 3 Feb 2011. Web. 23 Dec 2016. http://perfecthealthdiet.com/2011/02/hunter-gatherer-macronutrient-ratios-new-data/

65. "Estimated Calorie Requirements." WebMD. Web. 19 Dec 2016. http://www.webmd.com/diet/features/estimated-calorie-requirement.

66. Reinagel, Monica. "Is There an Optimal Ratio of PUFAs, MUFAs, and Saturated Fats?" Nutrition Over Easy. 30 May 2012. Web. 22 Dec 2016. http://nutritionovereasy.com/2012/05/is-there-an-optimal-ratio-of-pufas-mufas-and-saturated-fats/.

67. "Recommended Daily Intakes and Upper Limits for Nutrients." Consumer Lab. Web. 14 Dec 2016. http://www.consumerlab.com/RDAs/.

68. Bilsborough, Shane. "A Review of Issues of Dietary Protein Intake in Humans." International Journal of Sport Nutrition and Exercise Metabolism 16.2 (2006): 129-52. Web. 1 Jan 2017. https://www.ncbi.nlm.nih.gov/pubmed/16779921.

69. U.S. Department of Health & Human Services. "Iodine: Fact Sheet for Health Professionals." National Institutes of Health. 24 June 2011. Web. 14 Dec 2016. https://ods.od.nih.gov/factsheets/Iodine-HealthProfessional/.

70. Kresser, Chris. "Iodine for Hypothyroidism: Crucial Nutrient or Harmful Toxin?" Chris Kresser. 5 July 2010. Web. 13 Dec 2016. https://chriskresser.com/iodine-for-hypothyroidism-like-gasoline-on-a-fire/.

71. "Iodine." The World's Healthiest Foods. Web. 8 Oct 2017. http://www.whfoods.com/genpage.php?tname=nutrient&dbid=69.

72. Razaitis, Lynn. "The Liver Files." The Weston A. Price Foundation. 29 Jul 2005. Web. 11 Dec 2015. http://www.westonaprice.org/health-topics/the-liver-files/.

73. US Department of Agriculture, Agricultural Research Service: Nutrient Data Laboratory. USDA National Nutrient Database for Standard Reference, Release 28 (Slightly revised). Version Current: May 2016. Web. 1 May 2016. http://www.ars.usda.gov/ba/bhnrc/ndl.

74. Staggs CG, Sealey WM, McCabe BJ, et al. Determination of the Biotin Content of Select Foods Using Accurate and Sensitive HPLC / Avidin Binding. J Food Compost Anal 2004;17:767-76.

75. Institute of Medicine, Food and Nutrition Board. *Dietary Reference Intakes for energy, carbohydrate, fiber, fatty acids, cholesterol, protein and amino acids.* Washington (DC): National Academies Press; 2002.

76. Paddon-Jones D, Campbell WW, Jacques PF, Kritchevsky SB, Moore LL, Rodriguez NR, van Loon LJC.Protein and healthy aging. *Am J Clin Nutr* 2015;101(Suppl):1339S–45S.

77. Leidy HJ, Clifton PM, Astrup A, Wycherley TP, Westerterp-Plantenga MS, Luscombe-Marsh ND, WoodsSC, Mattes RD. The role of protein in weight loss and maintenance. *Am J Clin Nutr* 2015;101(Suppl):1320S–9S.

Made in the USA
Monee, IL
04 November 2026

67379772R00095